TAKING CHARGE OF YOUR FERTILITY

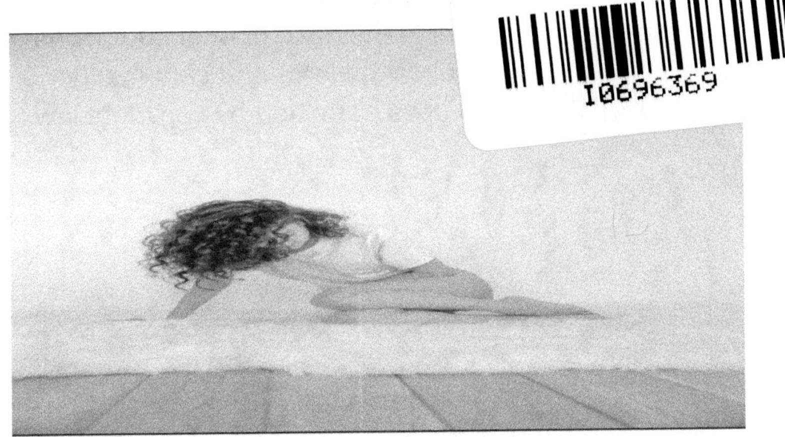

Empowering Women Through Knowledge: A Comprehensive Guide to Understanding and Navigating Your Fertility Journey

Emma Lynch

TABLE OF CONTENTS

INTRODUCTION

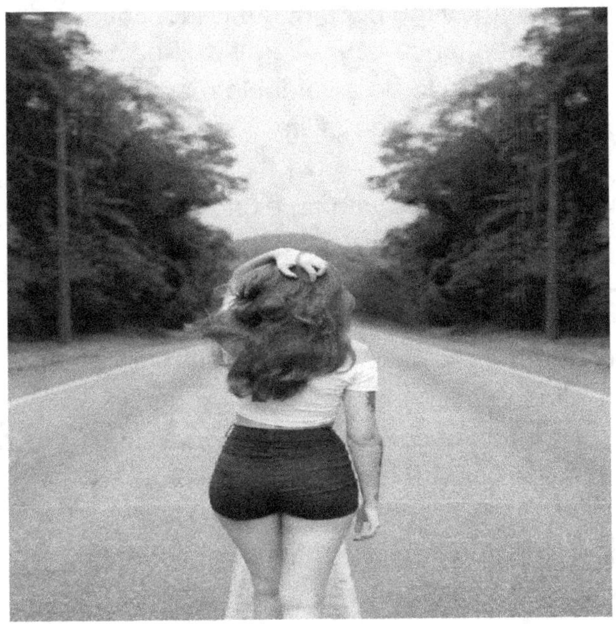

Embarking on the path of understanding and taking charge of your fertility marks a pivotal and empowering moment in your life. "Taking Charge of Your Fertility: A Comprehensive Guide" is designed as your companion in this journey, offering a wealth of knowledge and practical insights to empower you in making informed decisions about your reproductive health.

In the pages that follow, we will unravel the intricate nuances of the menstrual cycle, demystify the signs of ovulation, and explore the factors that influence fertility. Whether you are actively trying to conceive, seeking natural methods of contraception, or simply striving to enhance your overall well-being, this guide is crafted to be a valuable resource for women at every stage of life.

The journey begins with an exploration of the fundamentals—grasping the intricacies of your menstrual cycle and gaining a deeper awareness of the physiological markers that signify fertile and infertile phases. As we delve into the art of charting, recording basal body temperature, and interpreting the subtleties of cervical mucus, you'll find practical tools to decipher the language of your body.

Understanding fertility is not merely about conception; it's about embracing a holistic approach to reproductive well-being. We navigate through lifestyle factors, nutrition, and the impact of stress on fertility, empowering you with the knowledge to optimize your chances of conception or to maintain a healthy reproductive balance.

This guide also serves as a compass through the realm of contraception, presenting natural methods, barrier options, and medical alternatives. Whether you are actively planning for or against pregnancy, our goal is to provide you with a comprehensive understanding of your choices, allowing you to make decisions aligned with your personal values and goals.

Throughout this journey, we acknowledge the uniqueness of every woman's body and the various paths her fertility may take. Troubleshooting sections address common challenges, offering guidance on irregular cycles and when it might be time to seek professional advice.

Ultimately, this guide is not just about acquiring knowledge; it's about empowerment. We delve into advocating for personalized care, embracing the emotional and psychological aspects of your fertility journey, and moving forward with confidence and informed decision-making.

Welcome to "Taking Charge of Your Fertility: A Comprehensive Guide." May this resource serve as a beacon of knowledge, guiding you towards a deeper understanding of your body, fostering confidence in your choices, and empowering you to take control of your reproductive health.

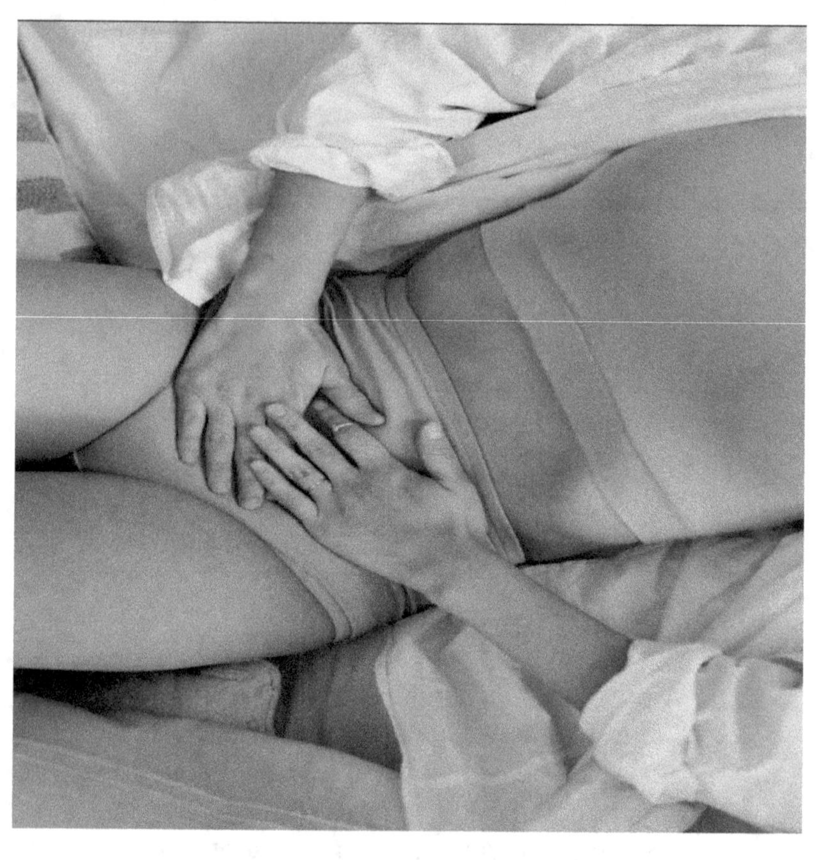

CHAPTER ONE

UNDERSTANDING YOUR MENSTRUAL CYCLE

The menstrual cycle is a complex and orchestrated series of events that occur in a woman's body, primarily governed by hormonal fluctuations. This cycle typically spans around 28 days, although variations are common. Here's a detailed breakdown of the key phases:

1. Menstruation (Days 1-5):
   - The cycle begins with menstruation, where the uterine lining, built up in the previous cycle, is shed if fertilization did not occur.
   - Estrogen and progesterone levels, among other hormones, are at their lowest.

2. Follicular Phase (Days 6-14):
   - The body moves into the follicular phase after menstruation.
   - The pituitary gland releases follicle-stimulating hormone (FSH), stimulating the ovaries to develop several ovarian follicles.
   - Each follicle contains an immature egg, but usually, only one becomes dominant.

- As this dominant follicle matures, it produces estrogen, which helps prepare the uterine lining for a potential pregnancy.
   - Estrogen levels rise, reaching a peak just before ovulation.

3. Ovulation (Around Day 14):
   - Ovulation marks the midpoint of the menstrual cycle and is triggered by a surge in luteinizing hormone (LH).
   - An egg that is ready for fertilization is released from the ovary by the dominant follicle.
   - This phase, lasting about 24-48 hours, represents the most fertile window for conception.

4. Luteal Phase (Days 15-28):
   - The burst follicle develops into the corpus luteum, a structure, following ovulation.
   - The corpus luteum produces progesterone, a hormone that maintains the uterine lining and prepares it for potential implantation of a fertilized egg.
   - If pregnancy does not occur, the corpus luteum degenerates, leading to a decline in progesterone levels.
   - The drop in hormone levels triggers the start of menstruation, and the cycle begins anew.

Understanding your menstrual cycle goes beyond a mere awareness of the phases. Charting additional signs such as basal body temperature, cervical mucus changes, and other bodily cues offers a more detailed and personalized insight into your fertility. This knowledge is not only valuable for those actively trying to conceive but also for those seeking a natural approach to contraception or simply aiming to connect more deeply with their bodies. By decoding the language of your menstrual cycle, you gain a powerful tool for navigating your reproductive health with informed decision-making.

BASICS OF FERTILITY AWARENESS

Fertility awareness is a valuable approach to understanding and managing your reproductive health. It involves tracking and interpreting various signs and symptoms throughout your menstrual cycle to identify fertile and infertile phases. Here are the basics:

1. **Basal Body Temperature (BBT):**
   - Tracking your basal body temperature, taken upon waking, helps pinpoint the shift that occurs after ovulation. When the temperature rises a little, ovulation has taken place.

2. **Cervical Mucus Changes:**
   - Observing changes in cervical mucus consistency provides insights into fertility. Around

ovulation, mucus becomes clear, slippery, and stretchy – resembling egg whites.

3. **Ovulation Prediction Kits (OPKs):**
   - The spike in luteinizing hormone (LH) that occurs prior to ovulation is detected by these kits. A positive result indicates a higher likelihood of ovulation within the next 24-48 hours.

4. **Menstrual Cycle Charting:**
   - Maintaining a menstrual cycle chart or calendar helps visualize patterns and identify fertile days. Note the start and end of menstruation, changes in cervical mucus, and positive OPK results.

5. **Tracking Menstrual Symptoms:**
   - Pay attention to physical and emotional changes throughout your cycle. Some women experience specific symptoms, such as breast tenderness or heightened libido, during fertile periods.

6. **Understanding Cycle Length:**
   - Consistent tracking allows you to determine your average cycle length. This knowledge aids in predicting when ovulation might occur and when to expect menstruation.

Fertility awareness is not only a tool for conception but also a natural method of contraception when used correctly. It empowers individuals to make informed choices about family planning, aligning with their unique goals and values. As you delve into the basics of fertility awareness, remember that consistency and keen observation are key to harnessing the full benefits of this approach.

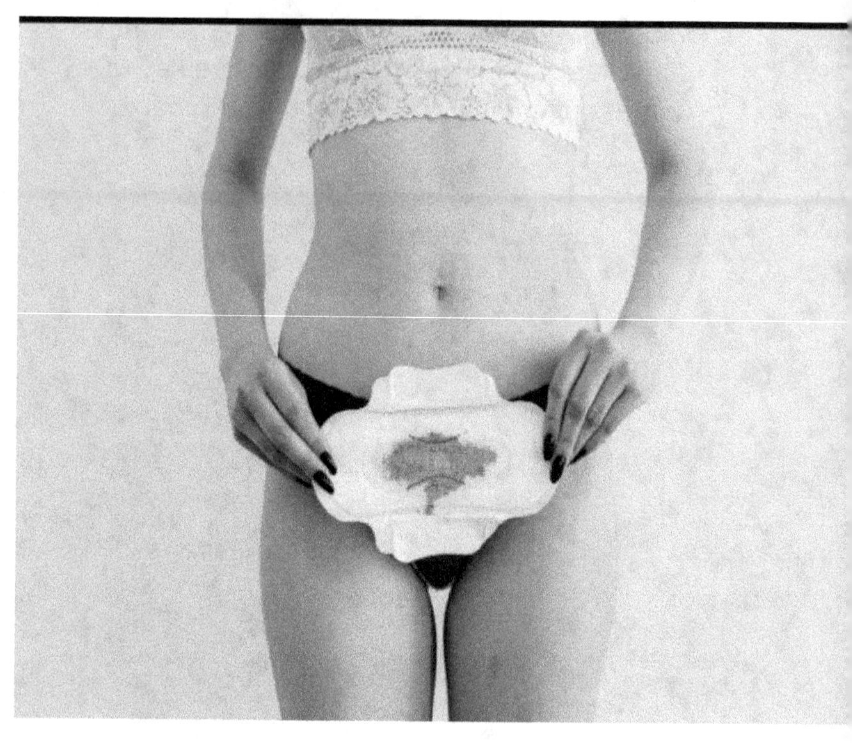

CHAPTER TWO

CHARTING YOUR CYCLE

Charting your menstrual cycle involves systematically recording various physiological changes throughout the month to gain insights into your fertility patterns. Here's a detailed explanation:

1. Establishing a Menstrual Calendar:
   - Start by creating a menstrual calendar to track the start and end dates of each menstrual cycle. Note the number of days your period lasts, as well as any irregularities or variations.

2. Basal Body Temperature (BBT) Charting:
   - Take a reading of your basal body temperature (BBT) before waking up each morning. Use a specialized basal thermometer for accuracy.
   - Record your temperature on a graph or chart. A slight increase in temperature (0.5-1.0°F) after ovulation indicates the end of the follicular phase.

3. Cervical Mucus Tracking:
   - Monitor changes in cervical mucus throughout your cycle. Begin by noting the sensation at the vulva and observing the mucus on toilet paper.
   - In the days leading up to ovulation, cervical mucus becomes clear, slippery, and stretchy – resembling egg whites. Record these changes on your chart.

4. Ovulation Prediction Kits (OPKs):
   - Use ovulation prediction kits (OPKs) to detect
the surge in luteinizing hormone (LH) that precedes
ovulation.
   - Mark positive OPK results on your chart, as they
indicate the fertile window, typically 24-48 hours
before ovulation.

5. Menstrual Symptoms and Sensations:
   - Record any physical or emotional symptoms
experienced during different phases of your cycle.
These could include breast tenderness, mood
changes, abdominal cramps, or increased libido.

6. Additional Observations:
   - Include other relevant information, such as
changes in lifestyle, stress levels, travel, or illness,
as these factors can influence your menstrual
cycle.

7. Regular Check-Ins and Analysis:
   - Regularly review your chart to identify recurring
patterns. Look for the consistent rise in BBT after
ovulation and note the length of your menstrual
cycles.
   - Some women may also observe secondary
fertility signs, like mittelschmerz (ovulation pain) or
changes in the cervix position.

8. Charting Apps:

- Utilize fertility tracking apps that allow you to input and analyze your data easily. These apps often provide predictions based on your recorded information and can streamline the charting process.

Benefits of Cycle Charting:
   - Enhanced fertility awareness for conception or natural contraception.
   - Identification of irregularities or potential health concerns.
   - Empowerment through a deeper understanding of your body's unique rhythm.

Remember, accurate charting requires consistency and patience. Over time, this practice can provide valuable insights into your fertility, empowering you to make informed decisions about family planning and reproductive health.

RECORDING BASAL BODY TEMPERATURE

Recording basal body temperature (BBT) is a key component of fertility awareness, offering valuable insights into the various phases of your menstrual cycle. Here's a detailed explanation of how to accurately record and interpret your BBT:

1. Understanding Basal Body Temperature (BBT):

- Basal body temperature refers to your body's temperature at rest, typically measured upon waking, before any physical activity, and even before getting out of bed.
   - This temperature reflects the metabolic changes associated with the menstrual cycle.

2. Choosing a Basal Thermometer:
   - Invest in a specialized basal thermometer with increased sensitivity (measuring temperature to two decimal places, e.g., 97.65°F).
   - Utilize a consistent thermometer to ensure precise measurements.

3. Establish a Routine:
   - Measure your BBT at the same time every morning, preferably before engaging in any physical activity, including sitting up or talking. The goal is to capture your body's lowest, resting temperature.

4. Consistency in Measurement:
   - Use the same method and location for each measurement. Oral measurements are common, but some women find vaginal or rectal measurements more accurate.
   - Ensure you've had at least three consecutive hours of sleep before taking your BBT.

5. Record the Temperature:
   - Record your temperature on a dedicated chart or in a fertility tracking app. Note any factors that

might affect the reading, such as illness, alcohol consumption, or poor sleep.

6. Detecting the BBT Shift:
   - Throughout the first part of your cycle (follicular phase), BBT remains relatively low. After ovulation, due to the influence of progesterone, there's a noticeable rise in BBT.
   - The temperature shift usually occurs 1-2 days after ovulation and remains elevated until the start of your next cycle.

7. Identifying Ovulation:
   - The BBT shift helps confirm that ovulation has occurred. Tracking it over several cycles helps pinpoint the most fertile days for conception.
   - Ovulation is generally recognized as the last day of lower temperatures before the rise.

8. Consider Additional Fertility Signs:
   - While BBT is a reliable indicator of ovulation, combining it with other fertility signs, such as cervical mucus changes and ovulation prediction kits, enhances the accuracy of fertility predictions.

9. Analyzing Your Chart:
   - Regularly review your BBT chart to identify patterns and trends. Understanding your unique cycle length and the timing of the BBT shift aids in predicting ovulation.

Recording basal body temperature is a meticulous but empowering practice, providing valuable information about your reproductive health. As you consistently chart your BBT over time, you gain a deeper understanding of your menstrual cycle, enhancing your ability to make informed decisions about family planning and fertility.

MONITORING CERVICAL MUCUS

Monitoring cervical mucus is a crucial aspect of fertility awareness, offering valuable insights into the various phases of your menstrual cycle. Here's a detailed explanation of how to accurately monitor and interpret cervical mucus changes:

1. Understanding Cervical Mucus:
   - Cervical mucus, produced by glands in the cervix, undergoes distinct changes throughout the menstrual cycle.
   - The consistency, color, and amount of cervical mucus are influenced by hormonal fluctuations, particularly estrogen.

2. Establish a Routine:
   - Begin monitoring cervical mucus from the first day of your menstrual cycle.
   - Consistency in the timing of observations is crucial, preferably at the same time each day.

3. Washing Hands:

- Ensure your hands are clean before collecting a sample of cervical mucus. This prevents contamination and provides accurate observations.

4. Observing Sensations:
   - Note any sensations at the vulva, as these can indicate the presence and type of cervical mucus. For example:
     - Dry or Sticky: No visible mucus, sensation of dryness or stickiness.
     - Creamy: Moist, white, or yellowish mucus, similar to hand lotion.
     - Egg White: Clear, stretchy, and slippery, resembling raw egg whites, indicating fertile days.
     - Watery: Thin, clear, and fluid, indicating increasing fertility.

5. Collecting Cervical Mucus:
   - Gently collect a sample of cervical mucus using clean fingers. Observe its color, texture, and stretchiness.
   - Stretch the mucus between your thumb and index finger to assess its elasticity. The more stretchy and clear it is, the more fertile the days.

6. Record Observations:
   - Record your cervical mucus observations on a dedicated chart or in a fertility tracking app. Note any additional factors like illness or medications that may influence mucus consistency.

7. Correlate with Menstrual Cycle Phases:

- Cervical mucus changes correlate with different phases of your menstrual cycle. Dry or sticky mucus is typical in the early follicular phase, while fertile cervical mucus appears leading up to and during ovulation.
   - After ovulation, cervical mucus often transitions back to a drier or stickier consistency.

8. Combine with Other Fertility Signs:
   - Combining cervical mucus observations with other fertility signs, such as basal body temperature (BBT) charting and ovulation prediction kits, enhances the accuracy of fertility predictions.

9. Personalized Understanding:
   - Every woman's cervical mucus pattern is unique. Regularly monitoring and understanding your pattern over several cycles is key to using this information effectively.

Monitoring cervical mucus provides a natural and reliable method for identifying fertile days, aiding both conception and natural contraception. As you become more familiar with your cervical mucus changes, you gain a deeper understanding of your reproductive health, enabling you to make informed decisions about family planning and fertility.

USING OVULATION PREDICTION KITS

Using ovulation prediction kits (OPKs) is a popular and effective method for identifying the fertile window within your menstrual cycle. These kits help predict ovulation by detecting the surge in luteinizing hormone (LH) that occurs approximately 24-48 hours before an egg is released from the ovary. Here's a detailed explanation on how to use OPKs:

1. Choose the Right Kit:
   - Purchase a reliable ovulation prediction kit. These kits typically include test strips or sticks that detect the presence of LH in your urine.

2. Determine When to Start Testing:
   - To pinpoint the best time to start testing, consider the average length of your menstrual cycle. Typically, ovulation takes place in the middle of your cycle.
   - For example, if you have a 28-day cycle, you might start testing around day 11 or 12.

3. Timing of Testing:
   - Test once a day, preferably in the afternoon, as LH levels typically surge in the morning and can take a few hours to appear in your urine.
   - Avoid excessive fluid intake for a couple of hours before testing to ensure more concentrated urine.

4. Read the Instructions:
   - Carefully read and follow the instructions provided with the OPK. Each kit may have specific guidelines for use.

5. Collecting Urine Sample:
   - Use a clean, dry cup or collect your urine midstream. Follow the kit instructions to either dip the test strip into the urine or use a provided container.

6. Interpreting Results:
   - Most OPKs have two lines – a control line and a test line. The test line becomes darker as LH levels rise.
   - A surge in LH is typically indicated by the test line becoming as dark as or darker than the control line.

7. Identifying the LH Surge:
   - Once the test detects an LH surge, ovulation is likely to occur within the next 24-48 hours.
   - Plan to have intercourse during this fertile window for the best chance of conception.

8. Consistency in Testing:
   - Test daily until you detect the LH surge, and continue for a few days afterward to ensure you don't miss the peak fertility period.

9. Tracking and Recording:
   - Record your test results on a fertility chart or in a dedicated app. This allows you to track patterns over multiple cycles.

10. Combining with Other Fertility Signs:

- Use OPK results in conjunction with other fertility signs, such as cervical mucus changes and basal body temperature charting, for a more comprehensive understanding of your fertility.

11. Understanding Cycle Variability:
   - Note that cycle length can vary, so it's essential to track your cycles over time to identify your unique pattern.

Using ovulation prediction kits can be an effective tool for couples trying to conceive or individuals tracking their fertility for natural contraception. By consistently and accurately using OPKs and understanding how they fit into the broader context of your menstrual cycle, you can enhance your ability to plan and manage your reproductive health effectively.

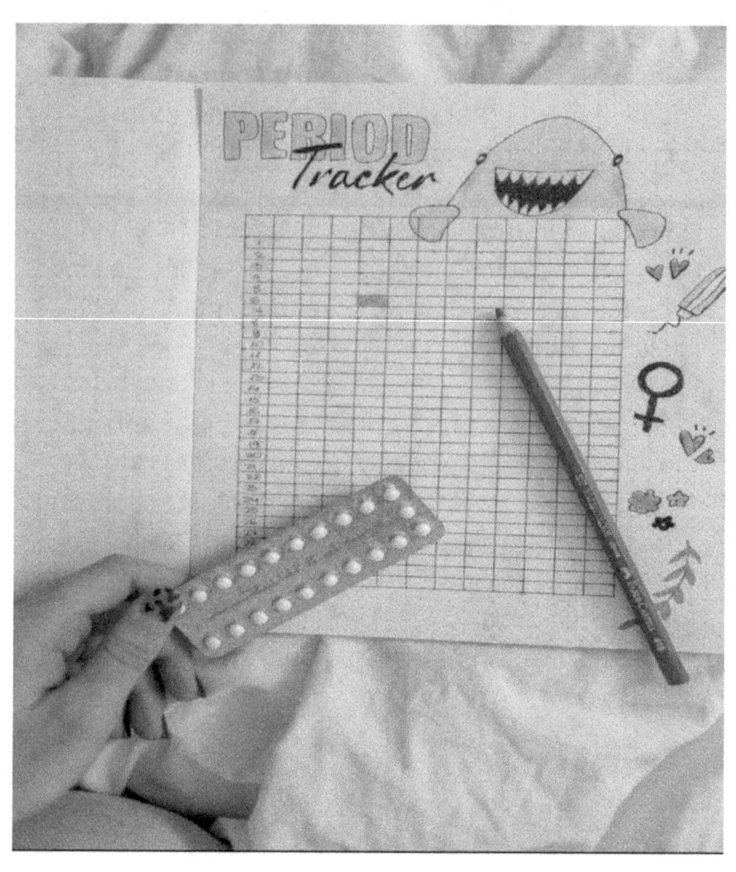

PERIOD
Tracker

CHAPTER THREE

INTERPRETING YOUR CHARTS

Interpreting your fertility charts involves analyzing the recorded data, such as basal body temperature (BBT) readings, cervical mucus changes, and other relevant observations, to gain insights into your menstrual cycle. Here's a detailed explanation:

1. Understanding Basal Body Temperature (BBT) Charts:
   - Start by reviewing your BBT chart. Identify patterns and trends over the course of your menstrual cycles.
   - Look for a distinct temperature shift. The increase in body temperature signifies the completion of ovulation.

2. Identifying the BBT Shift:
   - Ovulation typically causes a noticeable increase in BBT, usually around 0.5-1.0°F. This temperature shift persists through the luteal phase.
   - The day before the temperature rise is considered the likely day of ovulation.

3. Confirming Ovulation with Cervical Mucus:
   - Cross-reference BBT readings with cervical mucus observations. If you notice clear, stretchy mucus resembling raw egg whites, it aligns with the fertile window and confirms ovulation.

4. Consistency in Charting:
   - Consistency is key. Regularly charting your cycle over several months provides a more accurate understanding of your unique fertility patterns.

5. Analyzing Menstrual Symptoms:
   - Consider any physical or emotional symptoms recorded on your chart. Some women experience specific signs, such as breast tenderness or mood changes, correlating with certain phases of the menstrual cycle.

6. Correlating with Ovulation Prediction Kits (OPKs):
   - If using OPKs, note positive results on your chart. The LH surge detected by OPKs precedes ovulation by approximately 24-48 hours.

7. Tracking Cycle Length:
   - Pay attention to the length of your menstrual cycles. The time between ovulation and the start of the next menstruation constitutes the luteal phase, typically around 12-16 days.

8. Recognizing Regularity or Irregularities:
   - Assess the regularity of your cycle. Consistent patterns in the length of your follicular and luteal phases are indicative of a more predictable cycle.

- Irregularities, such as variations in cycle length or inconsistent BBT patterns, may warrant closer attention.

9. Seeking Professional Guidance:
   - If you observe persistent irregularities or have difficulty interpreting your charts, consider consulting with a healthcare professional or a fertility specialist for personalized guidance.

10. Combining Multiple Fertility Signs:
   - Integrating various fertility signs, including BBT, cervical mucus, and any other observed symptoms, provides a holistic view of your fertility.
   - Cross-referencing these signs enhances the accuracy of predicting fertile and infertile phases.

11. Empowering Informed Decision-Making:
   - Ultimately, the goal of interpreting your charts is to empower you with the knowledge to make informed decisions about family planning, whether you are trying to conceive or practicing natural contraception.

Interpreting your fertility charts is a skill that improves with consistent tracking and observation over time. By analyzing the interconnected signals your body provides, you gain a deeper understanding of your menstrual cycle, enabling you to navigate your reproductive health with confidence and precision.

IDENTIFYING FERTILE AND INFERTILE PHASES

Identifying fertile and infertile phases within your menstrual cycle is central to effective family planning, whether you're aiming to conceive or practicing natural contraception. Here's a detailed explanation:

1. Understanding Menstrual Phases:
   - Your menstrual cycle comprises distinct phases: the follicular phase leading up to ovulation and the luteal phase following ovulation.

2. Fertile Phase:
   - The fertile phase includes the days leading up to and around ovulation.
   - Ovulation is a key event; during this time, an egg is released from the ovary, and conception is most likely to occur.
   - The fertile window extends a few days before and after ovulation, encompassing the lifespan of both the egg and sperm.

3. Identifying Ovulation:
   - Techniques such as charting basal body temperature (BBT), monitoring cervical mucus changes, and using ovulation prediction kits (OPKs) help pinpoint ovulation.
   - The day of ovulation and the preceding days represent the peak fertility period.

4. Cervical Mucus Changes:
   - Observing changes in cervical mucus is a reliable method for identifying the fertile phase.
   - Stretchy, clear, and slippery cervical mucus resembling raw egg whites signifies increased fertility, creating an environment conducive to sperm survival and movement.

5. Ovulation Prediction Kits (OPKs):
   - Positive results on OPKs indicate the LH surge preceding ovulation. The fertile window typically spans 24-48 hours after a positive OPK result.

6. Timing Intercourse:
   - To maximize the chances of conception, engaging in sexual intercourse during the fertile window is crucial.
   - Sperm can survive in the female reproductive tract for several days, so having intercourse before ovulation contributes to the likelihood of fertilization.

7. Infertile Phase:
   - The infertile phase encompasses the days outside the fertile window.
   - Post-ovulation, the luteal phase begins, and the window of fertility closes until the next menstrual cycle.

8. Post-Ovulation Changes:
   - After ovulation, the body undergoes changes. Basal body temperature typically rises due to

increased progesterone levels, indicating the transition to the luteal phase.
   - Cervical mucus becomes less fertile, and the cervix returns to a firmer, less open state.

9. Charting for Confirmation:
   - Utilizing fertility charting methods, such as BBT and cervical mucus tracking, aids in confirming the transition from the fertile to the infertile phase.

10. Menstrual Cycle Regularity:
   - Regularity in menstrual cycle length contributes to more predictable identification of fertile and infertile phases.
   - Irregular cycles may present challenges, and professional guidance might be beneficial.

11. Natural Contraception:
   - For those practicing natural contraception, avoiding unprotected intercourse during the fertile window is a key strategy.
   - Understanding and respecting your unique fertility patterns are crucial for the effectiveness of natural contraception methods.

12. Seeking Professional Advice:
   - If conception challenges persist or if you have specific concerns about fertility, seeking guidance from a healthcare professional or fertility specialist is recommended.

Identifying fertile and infertile phases requires a combination of tracking methods and a nuanced understanding of your individual menstrual cycle. Regular and consistent charting, along with attention to additional fertility signs, empowers you to make informed decisions aligned with your family planning goals.

RECOGNIZING SIGNS OF OVULATION

Recognizing signs of ovulation is crucial for individuals trying to conceive or practicing natural contraception. Ovulation is the release of a mature egg from the ovary, and various physical and physiological changes can indicate this fertile period. Here's a detailed explanation:

1. Basal Body Temperature (BBT):
   - One important metric is basal body temperature. Before ovulation, your BBT is relatively stable. Following ovulation, due to the rise in progesterone, there is a noticeable and sustained increase in BBT.
   - Charting your daily BBT and identifying this temperature shift can help pinpoint ovulation, with the most fertile days being just before the temperature rise.

2. Cervical Mucus Changes:
   - Observing changes in cervical mucus is an effective method. As ovulation approaches,

estrogen levels rise, causing cervical mucus to become clear, stretchy, and slippery – resembling raw egg whites.
   - This fertile cervical mucus facilitates sperm movement and survival, indicating a prime time for conception.

3. Ovulation Pain (Mittelschmerz):
   - Some women experience ovulation pain or mittelschmerz, a mild twinge or cramping on one side of the lower abdomen. This usually happens at or near ovulation.

4. Cervical Changes:
   - The cervix undergoes changes during ovulation. As fertility increases, the cervix becomes softer, higher, more open, and produces more cervical mucus.
   - Performing regular cervical self-exams can help you recognize these changes.

5. Ovulation Prediction Kits (OPKs):
   - The spike in luteinizing hormone (LH) preceding ovulation is detected by OPKs. If the test is positive, ovulation is probably going to happen in the next 24 to 48 hours.

6. Increased Libido:
   - Some women experience an increase in libido or sexual desire during ovulation. This heightened interest in sex may be linked to hormonal changes.

7. Changes in Breast Sensation:
   - Hormonal fluctuations during ovulation can cause changes in breast sensitivity. Some women may have swelling or soreness in their breasts.

8. Mood Changes:
   - Ovulation can influence mood due to hormonal shifts. Some women report feeling more energetic, positive, or even experiencing a heightened sense of smell during this time.

9. Ovulation Spotting:
   - Ovulation spotting is light bleeding that can occur when the follicle ruptures to release the egg. It is typically a small amount of blood and may appear pink or brown.

10. Increased Ferning Patterns:
   - Using a fertility microscope to examine saliva for ferning patterns is another method. As estrogen levels rise, dried saliva under the microscope may exhibit fern-like patterns during the fertile phase.

11. Combining Multiple Signs:
   - Combining several of these signs enhances accuracy in identifying ovulation. For instance, noting BBT rise along with changes in cervical mucus and a positive OPK provides a comprehensive picture.

12. Regular Charting:

- Consistent charting and tracking of these signs over multiple cycles help establish patterns, allowing you to predict ovulation more accurately.

Recognizing signs of ovulation requires attentiveness to your body's cues and a commitment to consistent tracking. Whether your goal is conception or natural contraception, understanding these signs empowers you to make informed decisions about your reproductive health.

CHAPTER FOUR

FACTORS AFFECTING FERTILITY

Various factors can influence fertility, affecting an individual or a couple's ability to conceive. Understanding these factors is crucial for those trying to conceive or seeking to optimize reproductive health. Here's a detailed explanation of factors affecting fertility:

1. Age:
  - Female fertility declines with age, primarily due to a reduction in the quantity and quality of eggs. Fertility starts decreasing in the late 20s and accelerates after 35. Male fertility also declines with age, with a potential decrease in sperm quality and quantity.

2. Menstrual Cycle Irregularities:
  - Irregular menstrual cycles can indicate hormonal imbalances, impacting the regular release of eggs and making conception challenging.

3. Hormonal Imbalances:
  - Disorders such as polycystic ovary syndrome (PCOS) or thyroid dysfunction can disrupt hormonal balance, affecting ovulation and fertility.

4. Body Weight:
   - Conditions involving underweight or overweight people might affect fertility. Low body weight can lead to irregular menstrual cycles or amenorrhea, while obesity is associated with hormonal imbalances, insulin resistance, and ovulatory dysfunction.

5. Smoking and Substance Abuse:
   - Tobacco and recreational drug use, including excessive alcohol consumption, can adversely affect fertility in both men and women. Smoking, in particular, is linked to decreased ovarian reserve and sperm quality.

6. Nutrition and Diet:
   - Poor nutrition and unhealthy diet patterns can impact fertility. Deficiencies in essential nutrients such as folate, iron, and vitamins can affect reproductive health.

7. Stress:
   - Chronic stress can disrupt hormonal balance, potentially affecting ovulation and sperm production. For general well-being, learning efficient stress management skills is essential.

8. Sexually Transmitted Infections (STIs):
   - Untreated STIs can lead to pelvic inflammatory disease (PID) in women, causing scarring of the

fallopian tubes and increasing the risk of infertility.
STIs can impact the quality of sperm in men.

9. Environmental Factors:
   - Exposure to environmental pollutants, toxins,
and endocrine-disrupting chemicals can impact
fertility. Occupational exposures, such as those in
certain industries, may also play a role.

10. Structural Issues:
   - Structural issues in the reproductive organs,
such as blocked fallopian tubes, uterine fibroids, or
issues with the cervix, can hinder conception.

11. Genetic Factors:
   - Certain genetic factors can influence fertility.
Chromosomal abnormalities, such as those causing
conditions like Turner syndrome, can impact
reproductive health.

12. Medications and Medical Treatments:
   - Some medications and medical treatments,
such as chemotherapy and radiation, can affect
fertility. Certain medications may have side effects
impacting reproductive function.

13. Endometriosis:
   - Endometriosis, a condition where tissue similar
to the lining of the uterus grows outside the uterus,
can cause pelvic pain and interfere with fertility.

14. Male Factors:

- Sperm motility, count, and morphology are a few examples of the elements that can affect male fertility. Conditions like varicocele, hormonal imbalances, or genetic factors can affect male fertility.

Understanding these factors allows individuals and couples to take proactive steps in optimizing fertility. Seeking medical advice and addressing modifiable lifestyle factors can significantly improve the chances of successful conception.

LIFESTYLE AND NUTRITION

Lifestyle and nutrition play crucial roles in overall health, including reproductive health and fertility. Making positive choices in these areas can contribute to overall well-being and increase the likelihood of a healthy conception. Here's a detailed explanation:

1. Healthy Diet:
  - Adopting a well-balanced, nutritious diet is fundamental for reproductive health. A range of fruits, vegetables, nutritious grains, lean meats, and healthy fats should be included.
  - Ensure adequate intake of essential nutrients like folic acid, iron, calcium, and vitamins.

2. Weight Management:

- Fertility depends on maintaining a healthy weight. Both underweight and overweight conditions can negatively impact reproductive health.
   - Achieving and maintaining a healthy weight through a balanced diet and regular exercise can improve fertility outcomes.

3. Hydration:
   - Staying well-hydrated is important for overall health and can contribute to optimal fertility. Water helps in maintaining proper bodily functions, including those related to reproduction.

4. Limiting Processed Foods and Sugar:
   - Processed foods and excessive sugar intake can contribute to inflammation and hormonal imbalances, potentially impacting fertility.
   - Choose whole, unprocessed foods and limit the consumption of sugary beverages and snacks.

5. Regular Exercise:
   - Engaging in regular physical activity contributes to overall health, weight management, and stress reduction.
   - However, excessive exercise, especially in women, may negatively impact fertility, so maintaining a balanced exercise routine is crucial.

6. Stress Management:
   - Chronic stress can disrupt hormonal balance and ovulation, affecting fertility. Adopt stress

management techniques such as meditation, yoga, or deep breathing exercises.

7. Limiting Alcohol and Caffeine:
   - High alcohol and caffeine consumption has been linked to lower fertility. Moderation is key, and it's advisable to limit alcohol and caffeine consumption while trying to conceive.

8. Quitting Smoking:
   - Smoking is linked to decreased fertility in both men and women. Quitting smoking improves overall health and increases the chances of successful conception.

9. Adequate Sleep:
   - Getting enough sleep is essential for maintaining hormone balance and general health. Lack of sleep or irregular sleep patterns may affect reproductive hormones.

10. Avoiding Environmental Toxins:
   - Reduce your exposure to chemicals and pesticides, among other environmental pollutants. Choose organic produce when possible, and be mindful of personal care and household products.

11. Fertility-Boosting Nutrients:
   - There are some nutrients that are very good for fertility. For example, omega-3 fatty acids, found in fish and flaxseed, may support reproductive health.

12. Seeking Professional Guidance:
   - If you have specific concerns about nutrition and fertility, consider consulting with a healthcare professional or a registered dietitian specializing in reproductive health.

13. Preconception Planning:
   - Ideally, couples planning to conceive should engage in preconception planning. This involves adopting a healthy lifestyle, ensuring proper nutrition, and addressing any underlying health issues before conception.

14. Individualized Approach:
   - Since each person is different, what works for one may not work for another. Consider your individual needs, preferences, and any underlying health conditions when making lifestyle and nutrition choices.

Making positive lifestyle and nutrition choices is an investment in both reproductive health and overall well-being. By adopting a holistic approach to health, individuals and couples can enhance their chances of a healthy conception and pregnancy.

STRESS AND IMPACT

Stress can significantly impact overall health, and its effects extend to various aspects of well-being, including reproductive health and fertility.

Understanding the relationship between stress and its impact is crucial, particularly for individuals or couples trying to conceive. Here's a detailed explanation:

1. Stress and Hormonal Disruption:
   - Stress hormones like cortisol and adrenaline are released as a result of ongoing stress. Elevated levels of these hormones can disrupt the delicate balance of reproductive hormones, potentially affecting the menstrual cycle and ovulation.

2. Menstrual Irregularities:
   - Women experiencing chronic stress may encounter irregular menstrual cycles or even amenorrhea (absence of menstruation). Stress-related hormonal disruptions can affect the regularity of ovulation.

3. Impact on Ovulation:
   - Stress can inhibit the release of gonadotropin-releasing hormone (GnRH), a key regulator of the menstrual cycle. This, in turn, may suppress ovulation or lead to irregularities in the timing of ovulation.

4. Reduced Fertility:
   - Studies suggest that high levels of stress may reduce fertility by influencing the chances of conception. Stress-induced hormonal changes can affect the quality of cervical mucus and may interfere with the implantation of a fertilized egg.

5. Delayed Conception:
   - Couples experiencing high levels of stress may take longer to conceive compared to those with lower stress levels. Stress can contribute to suboptimal conditions for conception, affecting both male and female fertility.

6. Impact on Sperm Quality:
   - Stress can affect male reproductive health by influencing sperm quality. High stress levels have been associated with a decrease in sperm concentration and motility.

7. Increased Time to Pregnancy:
   - Couples dealing with chronic stress may experience a longer time to pregnancy. The interplay between stress, hormonal changes, and reproductive function can impact the overall fertility journey.

8. Impact on Libido:
   - Stress can reduce libido or sexual desire, impacting the frequency of intercourse and potentially affecting the chances of conception.

9. Assisted Reproductive Technologies (ART):
   - Stress may also influence outcomes in assisted reproductive technologies, such as in vitro fertilization (IVF). Some studies suggest that managing stress during fertility treatments may positively impact success rates.

10. Coping Mechanisms:
   - Individual responses to stress vary, and the effectiveness of coping mechanisms plays a role. Healthy coping strategies, such as mindfulness, meditation, or counseling, may mitigate the negative effects of stress on fertility.

11. Impact on Pregnancy:
   - Beyond conception, stress can also affect pregnancy outcomes. High levels of stress during pregnancy have been associated with preterm birth and low birth weight.

12. Addressing Underlying Issues:
   - Identifying and addressing underlying sources of stress, whether related to work, relationships, or lifestyle, is crucial. Counseling or treatment from a professional can be helpful.

13. Holistic Approach:
   - Taking a holistic approach to managing stress involves addressing physical, emotional, and lifestyle factors. This may include regular exercise, sufficient sleep, and activities that promote relaxation.

14. Seeking Professional Guidance:
   - Individuals or couples facing challenges with stress and fertility may benefit from seeking guidance from healthcare professionals, including

fertility specialists, who can provide personalized advice and support.

Recognizing the impact of stress on reproductive health underscores the importance of holistic well-being. Managing stress through healthy lifestyle choices, effective coping strategies, and seeking professional support can contribute to improved reproductive outcomes and overall fertility.

COMMON HEALTH ISSUES

Common health issues encompass a wide range of conditions that affect individuals across different demographics. Here's a well-detailed explanation covering some prevalent health issues:

1. Cardiovascular Diseases:
   - Cardiovascular diseases, including heart disease and stroke, remain leading causes of global morbidity and mortality. Risk factors include high blood pressure, high cholesterol, and lifestyle factors such as poor diet and lack of exercise.

2. Respiratory Conditions:
   - Respiratory issues, such as chronic obstructive pulmonary disease (COPD), asthma, and respiratory infections, impact millions globally. Smoking, air pollution, and occupational exposures contribute to these conditions.

3. Diabetes:
   - Type 1 and Type 2 diabetes both impair the body's capacity to control blood sugar levels. Lifestyle factors, genetics, and obesity contribute to the increasing prevalence of diabetes worldwide.

4. Mental Health Disorders:
   - Mental health issues, including depression, anxiety, and stress-related disorders, are widespread. Factors such as genetics, trauma, and societal pressures play a role in the development of mental health conditions.

5. Obesity:
   - Obesity is a global health concern associated with various health issues, including cardiovascular diseases, diabetes, and certain cancers. Poor diet, sedentary lifestyle, and genetic factors contribute to obesity.

6. Infectious Diseases:
   - Infectious diseases, ranging from the flu to more severe conditions like tuberculosis and HIV/AIDS, pose ongoing challenges. Vaccination, sanitation, and public health measures play critical roles in prevention.

7. Musculoskeletal Disorders:
   - Musculoskeletal issues, such as arthritis and back pain, affect a significant portion of the population. Aging, joint injuries, and sedentary lifestyles contribute to these conditions.

8. Cancer:
   - Cancer represents a diverse group of diseases characterized by uncontrolled cell growth. Risk factors include genetics, environmental exposures, and lifestyle choices such as smoking and poor diet.

9. Neurological Disorders:
   - Neurological conditions, including Alzheimer's disease, Parkinson's disease, and epilepsy, impact the nervous system. Age, genetics, and environmental factors contribute to the development of these disorders.

10. Gastrointestinal Disorders:
   - Gastrointestinal issues, such as irritable bowel syndrome (IBS) and gastroesophageal reflux disease (GERD), affect digestion and can significantly impact quality of life. Diet, stress, and genetic factors play roles in these conditions.

11. Reproductive Health Issues:
   - Reproductive health concerns encompass a range of issues, including infertility, polycystic ovary syndrome (PCOS), and sexually transmitted infections (STIs). Lifestyle, genetics, and access to healthcare influence reproductive health.

12. Allergies:
   - Allergic conditions, such as hay fever and food allergies, result from the immune system's

hypersensitivity to certain substances.
Environmental factors, genetics, and early
exposure play roles in allergy development.

13. Chronic Kidney Disease:
   - Chronic kidney disease affects the kidneys'
ability to filter blood effectively. Diabetes,
hypertension, and genetic factors contribute to the
development of kidney disease.

14. Autoimmune Disorders:
   - Autoimmune diseases, like rheumatoid arthritis
and lupus, occur when the immune system
mistakenly attacks the body's own tissues.
Genetics and environmental triggers are implicated
in autoimmune disorders.

15. Vision and Hearing Issues:
   - Vision and hearing impairments, including
conditions like cataracts and hearing loss, become
more prevalent with age. Genetics, environmental
exposures, and lifestyle choices contribute to these
issues.

Understanding these common health issues is
essential for individuals, healthcare professionals,
and policymakers to implement effective prevention
strategies, promote healthy lifestyles, and improve
overall public health outcomes. Addressing these
challenges requires a multifaceted approach
involving education, early detection, and access to
quality healthcare.

CHAPTER FIVE

CONTRACEPTION OPTIONS

Contraception, or birth control, involves the use of various methods to prevent pregnancy. There are numerous contraception options available, catering to different preferences, health considerations, and lifestyle choices. Here's a detailed explanation of some common contraception options:

1. Hormonal Methods:

  - **Oral Contraceptives (Birth Control Pills):**
    - These pills contain synthetic hormones (estrogen and/or progestin) that prevent ovulation, thicken cervical mucus, and alter the uterine lining. When taken regularly, they are very effective.

  - **Birth Control Patch:**
    - A tiny, sticky patch that is applied to the skin and delivers hormones to stop ovulation. It is typically changed weekly.

  - **Birth Control Ring:**
    - A flexible, hormonal ring inserted into the vagina, releasing hormones to prevent ovulation. It remains in place for three weeks, followed by a one-week break.

2. Long-Acting Reversible Contraception (LARC):

  - **Intrauterine Devices (IUDs):**
  - tiny, T-shaped implants placed inside the uterus. Progestin is released by hormonal IUDs, which delays ovulation and thickens cervical mucus. Copper IUDs create an environment toxic to sperm.

  - **Implants:**
  - Small rods placed under the skin of the upper arm. They release progestin, preventing ovulation and altering cervical mucus.

3. Barrier Methods:

  - **Male Condoms:**
  - Sheaths worn over the penis to prevent sperm from entering the vagina. They provide protection from STDs, or sexually transmitted infections.

  - **Female Condoms:**
  - Polyurethane pouches inserted into the vagina before intercourse, providing a barrier against sperm. Like male condoms, they also offer STI protection.

  - **Diaphragm and Cervical Cap:**

- Devices placed in the vagina before sex to cover the cervix and block sperm. Used with spermicide for increased effectiveness.

4. Emergency Contraception:

- **Emergency Contraceptive Pills (Morning-After Pills):**
- used to lower the risk of pregnancy during unprotected intercourse. They work by delaying ovulation or interfering with fertilization.

- **Copper IUD for Emergency Contraception:**
- An IUD can be inserted within a few days of unprotected sex to prevent pregnancy. It is a highly effective and longer-term emergency contraception option.

5. Natural Methods:

- **Fertility Awareness-Based Methods (FABMs):**
- Tracking menstrual cycles, basal body temperature, and cervical mucus changes to identify fertile days and avoid unprotected sex during that time.

- **Withdrawal (Pull-out) Method:**
- includes the man taking his penis out of his vagina prior to ejaculating. It is less effective than other methods and does not protect against STIs.

6. Sterilization:

  - **Tubal Ligation (Female Sterilization):**
    - A surgical procedure in which a woman's fallopian tubes are closed or blocked to prevent the egg from reaching the uterus.

  - **Vasectomy (Male Sterilization):**
    - A surgical technique that includes severing or obstructing the vas deferens to stop the release of sperm during ejaculation.

Choosing the most suitable contraception method depends on factors such as health, lifestyle, relationship status, and preferences. It's crucial to consult with healthcare professionals to discuss options, receive personalized advice, and ensure the chosen method aligns with individual needs and circumstances. Additionally, barrier methods are recommended for preventing STIs, and individuals with concerns about sexually transmitted infections should consider these factors when selecting a contraception method.

NATURAL METHOD

Natural methods of contraception, also known as fertility awareness-based methods (FABMs) or natural family planning, involve tracking and interpreting a woman's menstrual cycle to determine fertile and infertile phases. These methods are hormone-free and may appeal to individuals seeking non-invasive, natural approaches to family planning. Here's a well-detailed explanation of natural methods:

1. Tracking Menstrual Cycle:
   - FABMs involve tracking the menstrual cycle to understand the timing of ovulation, which is when an egg is released from the ovary and conception is most likely to occur.

2. Basal Body Temperature (BBT) Charting:
   - Basal body temperature is the body's resting temperature, and it typically rises slightly after ovulation due to increased progesterone levels. Charting daily morning temperatures helps identify the temperature shift indicating ovulation.

3. Cervical Mucus Observation:
   - Changes in cervical mucus throughout the menstrual cycle can signal fertility. Around ovulation, cervical mucus becomes clear, stretchy, and slippery, resembling raw egg whites. This fertile cervical mucus facilitates sperm movement.

4. Calendar-Based Methods:
   - Calculating fertile and infertile days based on the menstrual cycle length. The Standard Days Method identifies a fixed fertile window (days 8-19 in a 28-day cycle), while the Calendar Rhythm Method involves tracking cycle lengths over several months.

5. Symptothermal Method:
   - Combining multiple signs, such as BBT, cervical mucus, and calendar calculations, for increased accuracy in identifying fertile and infertile phases.

6. Ovulation Prediction Kits (OPKs):
   - Some FABM users incorporate ovulation prediction kits to detect the surge in luteinizing hormone (LH) that precedes ovulation. OPKs can provide additional confirmation of fertile days.

7. Standard Days Method (SDM):
   - Suitable for women with regular menstrual cycles of 26-32 days. It identifies a fixed fertile window (days 8-19) when conception is most likely.

8. TwoDay Method:
   - Based on observing cervical mucus. If any cervical mucus is noticed today or yesterday, the day is considered fertile.

9. Lactational Amenorrhea Method (LAM):
   - Temporary method suitable for breastfeeding mothers. The absence of menstruation during exclusive breastfeeding can be used to avoid pregnancy during the first six months postpartum.

10. Limitations and Effectiveness:
   - FABMs require consistent and accurate tracking, making them more suitable for individuals

with regular menstrual cycles who are willing to invest time and effort in monitoring fertility signs.

   - Effectiveness varies; perfect use can be highly effective, but typical use may result in higher failure rates.

   - They do not protect against sexually transmitted infections (STIs), so additional protection may be necessary if there is a risk of STI exposure.

11. Advantages:

   - Non-hormonal: FABMs do not involve the use of hormones, making them suitable for those who prefer hormone-free contraception.

   - Natural and Non-Invasive: FABMs rely on observing natural bodily signs without the need for devices or medications.

12. Disadvantages:

   - Requires Consistency: Success depends on consistent and accurate tracking, which may be challenging for some individuals.

   - Learning Curve: Mastering FABMs may take time, and there is a learning curve involved in correctly interpreting fertility signs.

13. Counseling and Education:

   - Individuals interested in natural methods should receive proper education and counseling. Professional guidance enhances the accuracy of tracking and interpretation.

Natural methods of contraception offer a hormone-free alternative for individuals who are comfortable with regular tracking and are motivated to understand and manage their fertility. It is essential to consult with healthcare professionals for guidance and support when considering these methods.

BARRIER METHODS

Barrier methods of contraception involve physical barriers that prevent sperm from reaching an egg, providing a reliable way to reduce the risk of pregnancy. These methods also offer some protection against sexually transmitted infections (STIs). Here's a well-detailed explanation of barrier methods:

1. Male Condoms:
   - **Description:** Thin sheaths typically made of latex, polyurethane, or polyisoprene, worn over the erect penis.
   - **How They Work:**
     - Make a physical wall that keeps sperm from passing through the vagina.
     - Collect and contain ejaculated semen.
   - **Effectiveness:**
     - When used correctly and consistently, male condoms are highly effective, providing a reliable barrier against both pregnancy and many STIs.

2. Female Condoms:
   - **Description:** Soft, loose-fitting pouches with a closed end and a flexible ring at each end.
   - **How They Work:**
      - Inserted into the vagina before sex to cover the cervix and line the vaginal walls.
      - Creates a barrier, preventing sperm from reaching the egg.
   - **Effectiveness:**
      - While less commonly used than male condoms, female condoms offer a similar level of effectiveness when used consistently and correctly.

3. Diaphragm:
   - **Description:** Dome-shaped device made of silicone or latex, inserted into the vagina before intercourse.
   - **How It Works:**
      - prevents sperm from entering the uterus by covering the cervix.
      - used in conjunction with spermicide to boost efficacy.
   - **Effectiveness:**
      - Effectiveness increases when used consistently and correctly with spermicide.

4. Cervical Cap:
   - **Description:** Thimble-shaped silicone or latex cap fitted onto the cervix.
   - **How It Works:**
      - keeps sperm from accessing the uterus by covering the cervix.

- Used with spermicide to enhance effectiveness.
  - **Effectiveness:**
    - Effectiveness increases with proper use and when used with spermicide.

5. Spermicides:
  - **Description:** Chemical substances available in various forms (creams, gels, foams, suppositories) that contain sperm-killing agents.
  - **How They Work:**
    - Kill or immobilize sperm, preventing them from reaching and fertilizing an egg.
    - Often used in conjunction with barrier methods like diaphragms or cervical caps.
  - **Effectiveness:**
    - While less effective on their own, spermicides can enhance the effectiveness of other barrier methods.

6. Advantages of Barrier Methods:
  - **Dual Protection:** Barrier methods offer protection against both unintended pregnancy and many STIs, making them a versatile choice for sexually active individuals.
  - **Readily Available:** Condoms, in particular, are widely available without a prescription and can be purchased at various locations.

7. Considerations and Tips:

- **Consistency is Key:** For optimal effectiveness, consistent and correct use of barrier methods is crucial.
  - **Allergy Considerations:** Individuals with latex allergies can use non-latex options like polyurethane or polyisoprene condoms.
  - **Sensitivity to Spermicides:** Some individuals may experience irritation or allergies to spermicides, and alternative methods may be considered.

8. Limitations:
  - **User-Dependent:** Effectiveness relies on proper and consistent use by both partners.
  - **Interrupts Spontaneity:** Some individuals may find the need to stop and use a barrier method disrupts the spontaneity of sexual activity.

Barrier methods provide a practical and accessible option for those seeking contraception and protection against STIs. Proper education on correct usage, consideration of individual preferences, and communication between partners are essential aspects of successfully incorporating barrier methods into a contraceptive plan.

MEDICAL OPTIONS

Medical options for contraception involve the use of medications to prevent pregnancy. These methods often utilize hormones to regulate the reproductive system and prevent ovulation. Here's a well-detailed explanation of some common medical options:

1. Birth Control Pills (Oral Contraceptives):
   - **Description:** Pills containing synthetic hormones (estrogen and/or progestin) that mimic the natural hormones in a woman's body.
   - **How They Work:**
      - Inhibit ovulation, preventing the release of an egg from the ovary.
      - thicken cervical mucus to hinder sperm from accessing the egg.
      - Modify the uterine lining to discourage implantation.
   - **Effectiveness:**
      - Extremely successful when taken appropriately and consistently.

2. Birth Control Patch:
   - **Description:** A small, thin patch worn on the skin, releasing hormones similar to those in birth control pills.
   - **How It Works:**
      - Prevents ovulation.
      - Thickens cervical mucus.
      - Alters the uterine lining.
   - **Usage:**
      - Applied once a week for three weeks, followed by a one-week break.

3. Birth Control Ring (Vaginal Ring):

- **Description:** A flexible, hormonal ring inserted into the vagina, releasing estrogen and progestin.
    - **How It Works:**
        - Inhibits ovulation.
        - Thickens cervical mucus.
        - Alters the uterine lining.
    - **Usage:**
        - placed there for three weeks, then taken a week off.

4. Injectable Contraceptives:
    - **Description:** Hormonal injections administered every few months.
    - **How They Work:**
        - Suppress ovulation.
        - Thicken cervical mucus.
        - Modify the uterine lining.
    - **Usage:**
        - Typically administered every 1 to 3 months.

5. Birth Control Implant:
    - **Description:** A small rod placed under the skin of the upper arm, releasing progestin.
    - **How It Works:**
        - Suppresses ovulation.
        - Thins the uterine lining.
        - Thickens cervical mucus.
    - **Usage:**
        - Provides protection for up to three years.

6. Emergency Contraceptive Pills:

- **Description:** High-dose hormonal pills taken after unprotected sex to prevent pregnancy.
  - **How They Work:**
    - Delay ovulation.
    - Interfere with fertilization.
    - May affect the uterine lining.
  - **Usage:**
    - must be taken as soon as feasible following unprotected sexual activity.

7. Intrauterine Devices (IUDs):
  - **Description:** Small, T-shaped devices inserted into the uterus.
  - **How They Work:**
    - Copper IUDs create a hostile environment for sperm, inhibiting fertilization.
    - Hormonal IUDs release progestin, preventing ovulation, thickening cervical mucus, and altering the uterine lining.
  - **Usage:**
    - Depending on the type, effective for three to ten years.

8. Benefits of Medical Options:
  - **Highly Effective:** When used consistently and correctly, medical options are highly effective at preventing pregnancy.
  - **Regularity and Predictability:** Many methods provide regular and predictable menstrual cycles, which can be beneficial for planning.

9. Considerations:

- **Prescription Requirement:** Most medical options require a prescription and should be prescribed by a healthcare professional.
- **Side Effects:** Some individuals may experience side effects, such as nausea, breast tenderness, or mood changes. These typically disappear within a few months.

10. Limitations:
- **No STI Protection:** Medical options do not protect against sexually transmitted infections (STIs). It could be required to use condoms or other extra precaution.

Choosing a medical option for contraception involves considering factors like overall health, lifestyle, and personal preferences. Consulting with a healthcare professional is crucial to determine the most suitable method based on individual needs and circumstances.

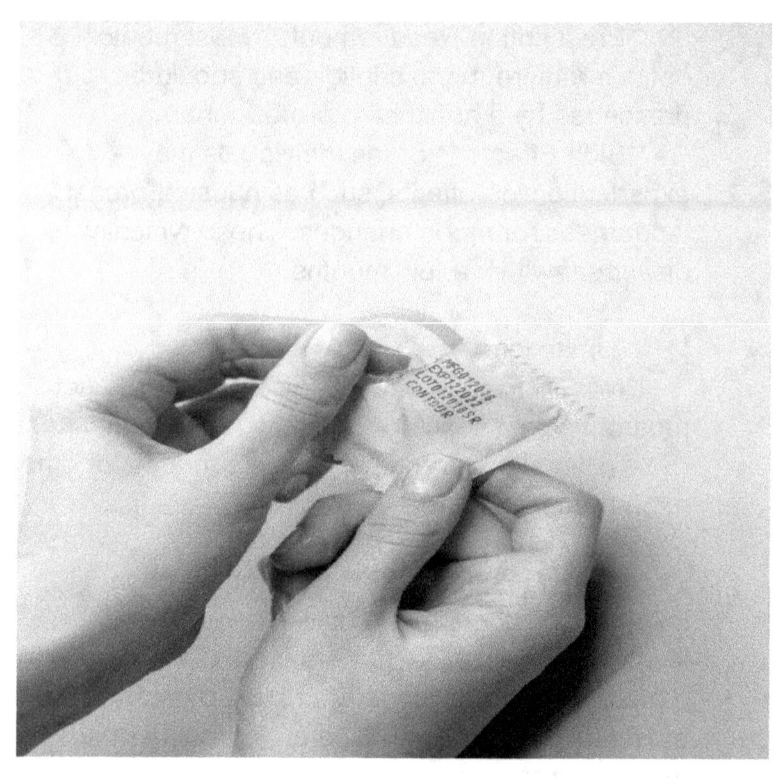

MFG01201
EXP122022
LOT01201BSR
CONTOUR

CHAPTER SIX

ACHIEVING PREGNANCY

Achieving pregnancy involves understanding the factors that influence fertility and implementing strategies to optimize the chances of conception. Here's a well-detailed explanation on achieving pregnancy:

1. Understanding Menstrual Cycle:
  - **Ovulation Awareness:**
    - Track the menstrual cycle to identify the fertile window when ovulation occurs. Ovulation usually happens around the middle of the menstrual cycle.

2. Basal Body Temperature (BBT) Charting:
  - **How It Works:**
    - Measure body temperature daily before getting out of bed.
    - An increase in body temperature signifies the completion of ovulation.
  - **Timing:**
    - The fertile window is typically a few days before the temperature rise.

3. Cervical Mucus Monitoring:
  - **How It Works:**
    - Observe changes in cervical mucus.
    - Fertile cervical mucus is clear, stretchy, and resembles raw egg whites.

- **Timing:**
    - Indicates approaching ovulation.

4. Regular Intercourse:
  - **Frequency:**
    - Aim for regular intercourse throughout the menstrual cycle, but particularly during the fertile window.
  - **Sperm Longevity:**
    - The likelihood of conception is increased by the fact that sperm can live for several days in the female reproductive system.

5. Healthy Lifestyle Choices:
  - **Balanced Diet:**
    - Maintain a nutritious and well-balanced diet to support overall health and reproductive function.
  - **Exercise:**
    - Engage in regular, moderate exercise to promote overall well-being.
  - **Avoid Excessive Alcohol and Tobacco:**
    - Limit alcohol intake and avoid smoking, as these can negatively impact fertility.

6. Maintain a Healthy Weight:
  - **Understand BMI:**
    - Fertility can be impacted by disorders like as underweight or overweight.
    - Achieving and maintaining a healthy weight is crucial for reproductive health.

7. Minimize Stress:

- **Impact of Stress:**
    - Chronic stress can affect hormonal balance and may interfere with ovulation.
    - **Stress Management:**
    - Adopt stress management techniques such as mindfulness, meditation, or yoga.

8. Preconception Health:
  - **Consultation with Healthcare Professional:**
    - Schedule a preconception checkup with a healthcare provider to address any existing health concerns.
    - Discuss any medications or conditions that may affect fertility.

9. Folic Acid Supplementation:
  - **Importance of Folic Acid:**
    - Begin taking folic acid supplements before conception to reduce the risk of neural tube defects in the developing fetus.

10. Timing of Intercourse:
  - **Frequency During Fertile Window:**
    - Aim for intercourse every 1-2 days during the fertile window.
    - Avoid placing excessive pressure on timing, as stress can negatively impact fertility.

11. Seek Professional Guidance:
  - **Consult a Fertility Specialist:**

- If conception does not occur after a year of regular, unprotected intercourse, consider seeking advice from a fertility specialist.
- Earlier consultation may be warranted for individuals over 35 or those with known fertility issues.

12. Monitor Men's Reproductive Health:
   - **Sperm Health:**
- Men should also maintain a healthy lifestyle, as sperm quality can impact fertility.
- If concerns arise, consider a semen analysis.

13. Fertility Treatments:
   - **Options:**
- In cases of prolonged infertility, fertility treatments such as in vitro fertilization (IVF) or assisted reproductive technologies (ART) may be considered.

14. Patience and Persistence:
   - **Realistic Expectations:**
- Conception may take time, and it's normal for healthy couples to take several months to achieve pregnancy.
- Patience and perseverance are essential during the process.

Optimizing the chances of achieving pregnancy involves a combination of understanding the menstrual cycle, adopting a healthy lifestyle, and seeking professional guidance when needed. Each individual's journey is unique, and consulting with healthcare professionals can provide personalized advice based on specific circumstances.

TIMING INTERCOURSE FOR CONCEPTION

Timing intercourse for conception involves understanding the woman's menstrual cycle, identifying the fertile window, and maximizing the chances of sperm meeting the egg. Here's a detailed explanation:

1. Menstrual Cycle and Ovulation:
   - Although it might vary, the menstrual cycle normally lasts for 28 days. Ovulation, the release of an egg from the ovary, usually occurs around the middle of the cycle.

2. Identifying the Fertile Window:
   - The time during the menstrual cycle when a woman is most likely to become pregnant is known as the "fertile window." It includes the days leading up to ovulation and the day of ovulation itself.

3. Menstrual Cycle Phases:
   - **Menstrual Phase (Days 1-5):**
      - The first day of menstrual bleeding is considered the start of the cycle.

   - **Follicular Phase (Days 6-14):**

- The ovaries develop follicles, and one matures, preparing for ovulation.

  - **Ovulation (Around Days 14-15):**
    - The mature egg is released from the ovary, entering the fallopian tube.

  - **Luteal Phase (Days 15-28):**
    - The remaining follicle transforms into the corpus luteum, releasing hormones to prepare the uterus for a potential pregnancy.

4. Calculating the Fertile Window:
  - **Regular Menstrual Cycles (28 days):**
    - The fertile window is typically around days 10-17 of the menstrual cycle, with ovulation around day 14.

  - **Irregular Menstrual Cycles:**
    - Ovulation may vary, and tracking additional signs like cervical mucus and basal body temperature can help pinpoint the fertile window.

5. Monitoring Cervical Mucus:
  - **Fertile Cervical Mucus:**
    - Becomes clear, stretchy, and slippery around ovulation, facilitating sperm movement.

6. Basal Body Temperature (BBT) Charting:
  - **Rise in BBT:**

- After ovulation, there is a slight rise in basal body temperature due to increased progesterone levels.

7. Predicting Ovulation:
   - **Ovulation Prediction Kits (OPKs):**
   - Seek out the spike in luteinizing hormone (LH) preceding the ovulation period.
   - Intercourse is recommended in the days following a positive OPK result.

8. Frequency of Intercourse:
   - **Regular Intercourse Throughout the Cycle:**
   - To ensure sperm availability during the fertile window, aim for regular intercourse every 1-2 days throughout the menstrual cycle.

   - **Increased Frequency During Fertile Window:**
   - During the fertile window, consider increasing the frequency of intercourse to every day or every other day.

9. Avoiding Stress:
   - **Impact of Stress:**
   - Stress can potentially affect fertility and the regularity of the menstrual cycle.
   - Implement stress-reducing activities to maintain a relaxed state.

10. Positions and Post-Coital Activities:
   - **No Specific Position:**

- While some suggest certain positions may increase the chances of conception, there is no conclusive evidence.
    - Lie down for about 15-20 minutes after intercourse to allow sperm to reach the cervix.

11. Lubricants:
  - **Sperm-Friendly Lubricants:**
    - If needed, use lubricants specifically designed to be sperm-friendly or mineral oil.

12. Patience and Persistence:
  - **Realistic Expectations:**
    - Conception may take time, and healthy couples may take several months to achieve pregnancy.
    - Throughout the procedure, persistence and patience are essential.

13. Seeking Professional Advice:
  - **Consultation with a Healthcare Professional:**
    - If concerns arise or conception does not occur after a year of regular, unprotected intercourse, consider consulting with a healthcare professional or fertility specialist.

Understanding the menstrual cycle, monitoring fertility signs, and timing intercourse during the fertile window are key elements in maximizing the chances of conception. Each couple's journey is unique, and seeking professional advice can provide tailored guidance based on individual circumstances.

MAXIMIZING FERTILITY POTENTIAL

Maximizing fertility potential involves adopting lifestyle habits and practices that support reproductive health. Here's a detailed explanation on strategies to enhance fertility:

1. Healthy Lifestyle Choices:
  - **Balanced Diet:**
    - Consume a nutritious and well-balanced diet rich in fruits, vegetables, whole grains, lean proteins, and essential nutrients like folic acid and antioxidants.
    - Maintain a healthy weight to support hormonal balance.

  - **Regular Exercise:**
    - Engage in regular, moderate exercise, which can help regulate hormones, improve circulation, and contribute to overall well-being.

  - **Hydration:**
    - Sip enough water each day to stay well hydrated.

  - **Limit Caffeine and Alcohol:**

- Moderate caffeine intake and limit alcohol
consumption, as excessive amounts can potentially
impact fertility.

- **Avoid Smoking:**
- Quit smoking, as it can adversely affect both
male and female fertility.

2. Understand Menstrual Cycle and Ovulation:
- **Menstrual Cycle Awareness:**
- Track menstrual cycles to identify regular
patterns and understand the timing of ovulation.

- **Basal Body Temperature (BBT) Charting:**
- Monitor basal body temperature to identify the
shift that occurs after ovulation.

- **Cervical Mucus Observation:**
- Recognize changes in cervical mucus,
especially the appearance of fertile cervical mucus
around ovulation.

- **Ovulation Prediction Kits (OPKs):**
- Use OPKs to detect the surge in luteinizing
hormone (LH) that precedes ovulation.

3. Timing Intercourse:
- **Regular Intercourse:**
- Aim for regular intercourse throughout the
menstrual cycle to ensure sperm availability.

- **Increased Frequency During Fertile Window:**

- During the fertile window (leading up to and including ovulation), consider increasing the frequency of intercourse.

4. Manage Stress:
   - **Impact of Stress on Fertility:**
   - Persistent stress can mess with the menstrual cycle and hormonal balance.
   - Implement stress-reducing techniques such as meditation, yoga, deep breathing, or relaxation exercises.

5. Maintain a Healthy Environment:
   - **Avoid Environmental Toxins:**
   - Minimize exposure to environmental toxins and pollutants that may impact fertility.
   - Be cautious with certain occupational exposures and chemicals.

6. Men's Reproductive Health:
   - **Healthy Lifestyle for Men:**
   - Men should also adopt a healthy lifestyle, including a balanced diet, regular exercise, and avoidance of smoking and excessive alcohol.

   - **Limit Heat Exposure:**
   - Men should avoid prolonged exposure to excessive heat, such as hot baths or saunas, as it can affect sperm production.

   - **Limit Tight Clothing:**

  - Tight underwear or clothing that increases scrotal temperature should be avoided.

7. Preconception Health:
   - **Consultation with Healthcare Professional:**
     - Make an appointment for a healthcare provider's preconception checkup.
     - Discuss any existing health conditions, medications, or concerns related to fertility.

   - **Folic Acid Supplementation:**
     - Begin taking folic acid supplements before conception to reduce the risk of neural tube defects in the developing fetus.

8. Seeking Professional Advice:
   - **Consultation with a Fertility Specialist:**
     - If concerns arise or conception does not occur after a year of regular, unprotected intercourse, consider consulting with a fertility specialist.
     - Earlier consultation may be warranted for individuals over 35 or those with known fertility issues.

9. Be Patient and Persistent:
   - **Realistic Expectations:**
     - Understand that achieving pregnancy may take time, and it's normal for healthy couples to take several months.
     - Maintain patience and persistence during the process.

Adopting a holistic approach to health and well-being, along with understanding and monitoring fertility signs, can contribute to maximizing fertility potential. It's essential for both partners to actively participate in lifestyle adjustments and seek professional guidance when needed.

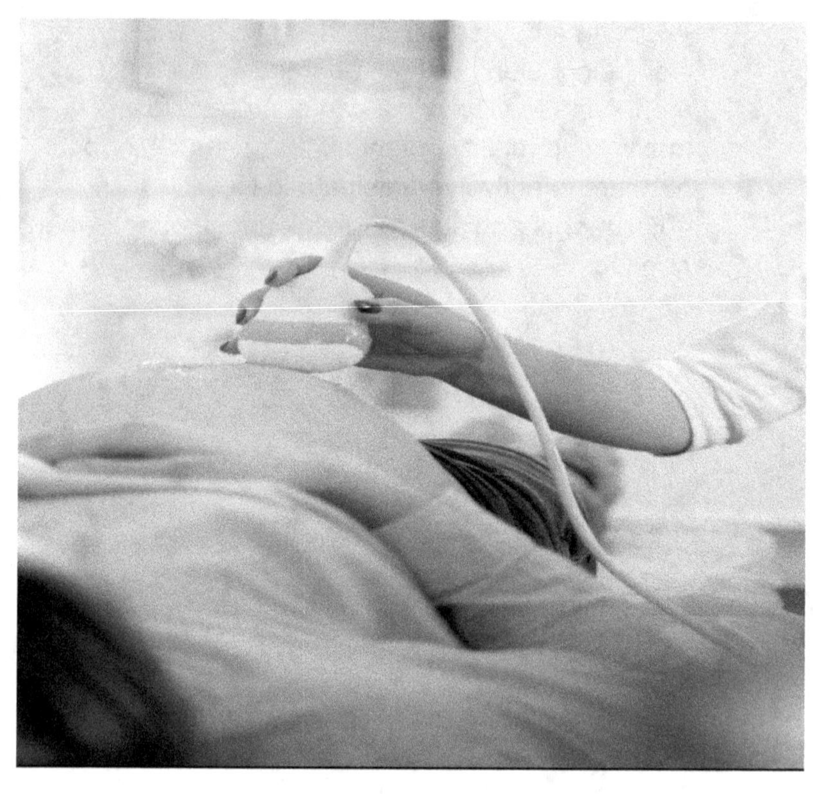

CHAPTER SEVEN

TROUBLESHOOTING

Troubleshooting fertility issues involves identifying potential factors that may impact conception and taking steps to address or mitigate them. Here's a detailed explanation on troubleshooting fertility concerns:

1. Understanding the Basics:
   - **Normal Conception Timeframe:**
     - Healthy couples can expect to wait up to a year to conceive.
     - If pregnancy does not occur within this timeframe, it may be time to explore potential issues.

2. Monitor Menstrual Cycles and Ovulation:
   - **Irregular Menstrual Cycles:**
     - Identify irregularities in menstrual cycles, as irregularities can impact ovulation.
     - Use methods like basal body temperature (BBT) charting, ovulation prediction kits (OPKs), and cervical mucus monitoring to track ovulation.

3. Health Assessment:
   - **Preconception Health Checkup:**
     - Schedule a preconception health checkup with a healthcare provider.

- Discuss existing health conditions, medications, and lifestyle factors that may affect fertility.

  - **Men's Reproductive Health:**
    - Consider a semen analysis for men to assess sperm count, motility, and morphology.

4. Lifestyle Factors:
  - **Review Lifestyle Choices:**
    - Evaluate diet, exercise, and overall lifestyle habits.
    - Address factors such as excessive caffeine or alcohol intake, smoking, and high stress levels.

  - **Weight Management:**
    - Achieve and maintain a healthy weight, as both underweight and overweight conditions can impact fertility.

  - **Environmental Toxins:**
    - Minimize exposure to environmental toxins and pollutants that may affect reproductive health.

5. Sexual Practices:
  - **Timing Intercourse:**
    - Reassess the timing of intercourse during the menstrual cycle, ensuring regular and increased frequency during the fertile window.

  - **Avoid Lubricants That Can Affect Sperm:**

- Some lubricants can impair sperm motility. Consider using sperm-friendly lubricants or mineral oil.

6. Stress Management:
   - **Impact of Stress on Fertility:**
   - Evaluate stress levels and consider stress-reduction techniques such as meditation, yoga, or counseling.

7. Medical Conditions:
   - **Identify and Address Medical Conditions:**
   - Certain medical conditions, such as polycystic ovary syndrome (PCOS) or endometriosis, can affect fertility.
   - Treatment plans, medications, or procedures may be recommended based on the specific condition.

8. Hormonal Imbalances:
   - **Hormone Testing:**
   - Consider hormone testing to identify any hormonal imbalances that may impact fertility.
   - Addressing hormonal issues may involve medications or lifestyle adjustments.

9. Age-Related Factors:
   - **Consider Age Factors:**
   - Age can impact fertility, particularly for women over 35.
   - If concerns persist, seek guidance from a fertility specialist.

10. Male Fertility Issues:
  - **Semen Analysis:**
    - If conception is delayed, a semen analysis for the male partner can provide insights into sperm health.

  - **Urologist Consultation:**
    - If issues are identified, consult with a urologist or fertility specialist for further evaluation and guidance.

11. Fertility Treatments:
  - **Consult a Fertility Specialist:**
    - If troubleshooting efforts do not yield results, consider consulting a fertility specialist.
    - Assisted reproductive technologies (ART) or fertility treatments may be explored.

12. Emotional Support:
  - **Counseling or Support Groups:**
    - Infertility can be emotionally challenging. Seek counseling or join support groups to cope with the emotional aspects of the journey.

Troubleshooting fertility issues involves a comprehensive approach, addressing both physical and emotional factors. Seeking professional advice, maintaining open communication with healthcare providers, and exploring available resources for emotional support can contribute to a more informed and empowered journey toward conception.

ADDRESSING IRREGULAR CYCLES

Addressing irregular menstrual cycles involves understanding the underlying causes and implementing strategies to regulate the menstrual cycle. Here's a well-detailed explanation on how to address irregular cycles:

1. Identify the Underlying Causes:
   - **Hormonal Imbalances:**
     - Hormonal fluctuations, such as those related to polycystic ovary syndrome (PCOS) or thyroid disorders, can cause irregular cycles.
   - **Stress:**
     - Chronic stress can impact the hypothalamus and disrupt normal hormonal signaling, leading to irregular cycles.
   - **Weight Changes:**
     - Rapid weight loss or gain can affect hormone levels and menstrual regularity.
   - **Medical Conditions:**
     - Certain medical conditions, such as uterine fibroids or endometriosis, may contribute to irregular cycles.

2. Seek Professional Guidance:
   - **Consult with a Healthcare Provider:**

- Schedule a consultation with a healthcare provider to discuss irregular cycles.
    - Provide detailed information about cycle lengths, symptoms, and any potential contributing factors.

  - **Hormone Testing:**
    - Hormone tests, including thyroid function tests and reproductive hormone levels, may be recommended to identify hormonal imbalances.

  - **Pelvic Examination:**
    - A pelvic examination or imaging studies may be conducted to assess for conditions like fibroids or endometriosis.

3. Lifestyle Modifications:
  - **Maintain a Healthy Weight:**
    - A healthy weight can be attained and maintained with a well-balanced diet and frequent exercise.
    - See a dietitian or other medical professional for individualized advice.

  - **Stress Management:**
    - Include stress-relieving exercises like yoga, mindfulness, or meditation.
    - Ensure adequate sleep and prioritize self-care.

  - **Regular Exercise:**

- Engage in regular, moderate exercise, which can help regulate hormonal balance.

- **Avoid Excessive Caffeine and Alcohol:**
- Limit caffeine intake and avoid excessive alcohol consumption, as these can contribute to hormonal disruptions.

4. Medications:
- **Hormonal Contraceptives:**
- Birth control pills or hormonal contraceptives may be prescribed to regulate menstrual cycles.
- These medications can help regulate hormonal fluctuations and induce regular, predictable cycles.

- **Metformin (for PCOS):**
- In cases of PCOS, medications like metformin may be prescribed to address insulin resistance and regulate menstrual cycles.

5. Addressing Underlying Conditions:
- **Treatment for PCOS:**
- Lifestyle modifications, medications, and fertility treatments may be recommended for individuals with PCOS.

- **Surgical Interventions:**
- In cases of conditions like uterine fibroids or endometriosis, surgical interventions may be considered to improve cycle regularity.

6. Fertility Awareness and Tracking:
   - **Basal Body Temperature (BBT) Charting:**
     - Monitoring BBT can provide insights into ovulation patterns and help identify irregularities.

   - **Ovulation Prediction Kits (OPKs):**
     - OPKs can help predict ovulation and identify the fertile window.

   - **Cervical Mucus Monitoring:**
     - Changes in cervical mucus can indicate approaching ovulation.

7. Follow-Up and Monitoring:
   - **Regular Checkups:**
     - Schedule regular follow-up appointments with the healthcare provider to monitor progress.
     - Adjust treatment plans or interventions as needed.

   - **Fertility Specialist Consultation:**
     - If irregular cycles persist or fertility concerns arise, consider consulting with a fertility specialist for more in-depth evaluation and guidance.

8. Patience and Persistence:
   - **Realistic Expectations:**
     - Addressing irregular cycles may take time, and changes may not happen overnight.
     - Maintain your patience and perseverance during the procedure.

Addressing irregular cycles involves a combination of lifestyle modifications, medical interventions, and tracking menstrual patterns. Seeking professional guidance is crucial to identify the specific causes and tailor a comprehensive plan for regulating menstrual cycles and promoting overall reproductive health.

SEEKING PROFESSIONAL ADVICE

Seeking professional advice for fertility concerns is a crucial step toward understanding and addressing potential issues. Here's a detailed explanation on how to navigate the process of seeking professional advice:

1. Initial Consultation:
   - **Choose a Healthcare Provider:**
   - Begin by scheduling an appointment with a healthcare provider, such as a gynecologist, reproductive endocrinologist, or a primary care physician.
   - Select a professional with expertise in reproductive health and fertility.

   - **Gather Relevant Information:**
   - Before the appointment, gather information about your medical history, menstrual cycle details, lifestyle factors, and any concerns you may have.

2. Preconception Checkup:

- **Comprehensive Health Assessment:**
    - During the initial consultation, expect a thorough health assessment to identify any existing medical conditions that may affect fertility.

  - **Discussion of Lifestyle Factors:**
     - Healthcare providers may inquire about diet, exercise, stress levels, and any habits that could impact fertility.

  - **Hormone Testing:**
     - Hormone tests, including those for thyroid function and reproductive hormones, may be ordered to assess hormonal balance.

  - **Pelvic Examination:**
     - A pelvic examination may be conducted to check for any physical abnormalities.

3. Male Partner Involvement:
   - **Semen Analysis:**
     - If applicable, the male partner may undergo a semen analysis to assess sperm count, motility, and morphology.

   - **Health Assessment for Men:**
     - Men may also be asked about lifestyle factors, medical history, and any concerns related to reproductive health.

4. Fertility Specialist Consultation:
   - **Referral if Needed:**

- If initial assessments indicate the need for specialized care, the healthcare provider may refer you to a fertility specialist or reproductive endocrinologist.

  - **In-Depth Evaluation:**
    - Fertility specialists conduct more in-depth evaluations, including advanced tests and imaging studies if necessary.
    - They specialize in identifying and addressing specific fertility issues.

5. Advanced Testing and Procedures:
  - **Hysterosalpingogram (HSG):**
    - This test involves injecting contrast dye into the uterus to assess the shape of the uterus and the patency of the fallopian tubes.

  - **Sonohysterography:**
    - An ultrasound procedure to evaluate the uterus and detect abnormalities.

  - **Ovulatory Function Tests:**
    - Advanced tests may be conducted to assess ovulatory function and identify potential issues.

  - **Genetic Testing:**
    - Genetic testing may be recommended if there is a history of genetic disorders or recurrent pregnancy loss.

6. Discussion of Treatment Options:

- **Tailored Treatment Plans:**
    - Based on the findings, the healthcare provider or fertility specialist will discuss tailored treatment options.
    - This may include lifestyle modifications, medications, assisted reproductive technologies (ART), or surgical interventions.

7. Emotional Support:
  - **Counseling Services:**
    - Recognize the emotional impact of fertility concerns, and consider seeking counseling or support groups for emotional well-being.

  - **Open Communication:**
    - Maintain open communication with the healthcare provider, expressing concerns, questions, and preferences regarding the treatment plan.

8. Second Opinion:
  - **Consider Seeking a Second Opinion:**
    - If unsure about the recommended treatment plan or diagnosis, consider seeking a second opinion from another qualified specialist.

9. Regular Follow-Up:
  - **Ongoing Monitoring:**
    - Regular follow-up appointments are essential to monitor progress, adjust treatment plans as needed, and address any new concerns.

10. Patience and Persistence:
  - **Understand the Process:**
    - Fertility treatment can be a journey, and success may take time.
    - Maintain patience, stay informed, and be persistent in following the recommended steps.

Seeking professional advice is a proactive and essential step in addressing fertility concerns. The collaborative efforts between healthcare providers, specialists, and patients contribute to a more informed and effective approach to fertility evaluation and treatment.

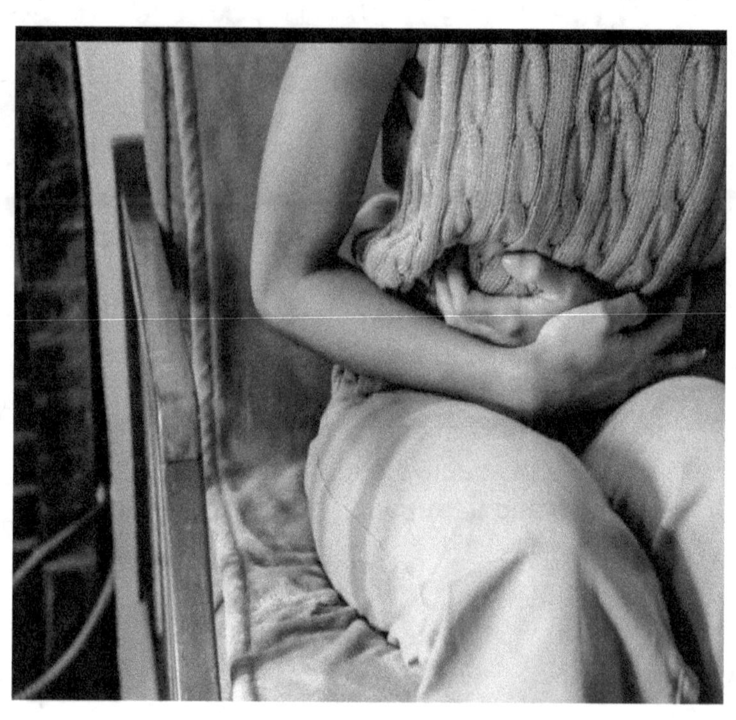

CHAPTER EIGHT

EMPOWERING YOUR REPRODUCTIVE HEALTH

Empowering your reproductive health involves taking proactive steps to understand, prioritize, and enhance your overall reproductive well-being. Here's a detailed explanation on how to empower your reproductive health:

1. Education and Awareness:
   - **Understand Your Body:**
     - Educate yourself about the anatomy and physiology of the reproductive system.
     - Learn about the menstrual cycle, ovulation, and factors influencing fertility.

   - **Stay Informed:**
     - Stay updated on reproductive health topics, advancements in fertility treatments, and overall wellness practices.

2. Regular Health Checkups:
   - **Schedule Routine Checkups:**
     - Visit your healthcare provider for regular gynecological checkups, including Pap smears, pelvic exams, and breast examinations.

   - **Preconception Health Checkup:**

- If planning to conceive, schedule a preconception health checkup to address any potential concerns and optimize your health before pregnancy.

3. Understand Your Menstrual Cycle:
  - **Track Menstrual Cycles:**
    - Keep a menstrual cycle diary or use apps to track your periods, noting cycle length, symptoms, and any irregularities.

  - **Learn About Ovulation:**
    - Understand the signs of ovulation, such as changes in cervical mucus and basal body temperature.

4. Lifestyle and Nutrition:
  - **Adopt a Healthy Lifestyle:**
    - Maintain a balanced diet rich in nutrients that support reproductive health, including folic acid, iron, and antioxidants.

  - **Regular Exercise:**
    - Engage in regular, moderate exercise to support overall well-being and hormonal balance.

  - **Limit Stress:**
    - Implement stress-management techniques such as meditation, yoga, or mindfulness to reduce the impact of stress on reproductive health.

  - **Avoid Harmful Substances:**

- Limit alcohol intake, avoid smoking, and minimize exposure to environmental toxins to protect reproductive health.

5. Fertility Awareness Methods:
   - **Basal Body Temperature (BBT) Charting:**
     - Use BBT charting to identify ovulation patterns and fertile windows.

   - **Cervical Mucus Monitoring:**
     - Pay attention to changes in cervical mucus to determine fertile periods.

   - **Ovulation Prediction Kits (OPKs):**
     - Use OPKs to predict ovulation and plan accordingly if trying to conceive.

6. Understand Birth Control Options:
   - **Educate Yourself:**
     - If not trying to conceive, understand various birth control options and choose the method that aligns with your reproductive goals and lifestyle.

7. Fertility Preservation:
   - **Consider Future Goals:**
     - If family planning is in the future, explore options for fertility preservation, especially if facing medical treatments that may impact fertility.

8. Emotional Well-Being:
   - **Acknowledge Emotions:**

- Recognize and address the emotional aspects of reproductive health, whether dealing with fertility challenges or family planning decisions.

  - **Seek Support:**
    - Consider seeking support from friends, family, or professionals to navigate emotional challenges and maintain overall well-being.

9. Stay Proactive:
  - **Advocate for Yourself:**
    - Be an advocate for your reproductive health by actively participating in discussions with healthcare providers, asking questions, and expressing your concerns.

  - **Second Opinions:**
    - If uncertain about a diagnosis or treatment plan, consider seeking a second opinion from another qualified specialist.

10. Fertility Specialist Consultation:
  - **Proactive Steps:**
    - If facing challenges in conceiving, consider consulting a fertility specialist early in the process.
    - Explore available fertility treatments and options.

11. Knowledge Sharing:
  - **Educate Others:**

- Share knowledge about reproductive health with friends and family to create awareness and reduce stigma surrounding fertility topics.

Empowering your reproductive health involves a holistic approach, combining knowledge, lifestyle choices, emotional well-being, and proactive healthcare practices. By taking an active role in understanding and prioritizing your reproductive health, you can make informed decisions and positively influence your overall well-being.

ADVOCATING FOR YOUR WELLBEING

Advocating for your well-being is a proactive and empowered approach to ensuring that your physical, mental, and emotional needs are met. Here's a detailed explanation on how to advocate for your well-being:

1. Self-Reflection:
   - **Know Your Needs:**
   - Consider your physical, mental, and emotional requirements.
   - Determine where you may require assistance or improvement.

2. Open Communication:
   - **Express Your Needs:**

- Practice open and honest communication with yourself and others.
- Express your demands, boundaries, and expectations clearly.

- **Seek Clarification:**
- If unsure about a situation or decision, ask for clarification.
- Obtain knowledge in order to make informed decisions.

3. Set Boundaries:
  - **Define Your Limits:**
- Define your personal and professional limits clearly.
- Set and maintain these boundaries in a courteous yet forceful manner.

  - **Learn to Say No:**
- Never be scared to say no when it's necessary.
- Put your health first and try not to take on more than you can handle.

4. Prioritize Self-Care:
  - **Make Time for Yourself:**
- Make self-care activities that support your mental, emotional, and physical health a priority.
- Schedule regular breaks and downtime.

  - **Acknowledge Burnout Signs:**

- Be aware of signs of burnout, stress, or fatigue.
- Take proactive measures to address these signs, such as seeking support or adjusting your workload.

5. Advocate in Healthcare:
   - **Ask Questions:**
   - During medical appointments, ask questions about your health, diagnoses, and treatment options.
   - Ask questions about any doubts or worries you may have.

   - **Seek Second Opinions:**
   - If facing a significant health decision, consider seeking a second opinion.
   - Ensure you are comfortable and fully informed about your health choices.

6. Mental Health Advocacy:
   - **Destigmatize Mental Health:**
   - Promote destigmatizing and raising awareness of mental health issues.

   - **Seek Professional Help:**
   - If experiencing mental health challenges, seek the help of mental health professionals.
   - Be an advocate for your own mental health by actively participating in the therapeutic process.

7. Education and Information:

  - **Stay Informed:**
    - Educate yourself on topics related to your well-being, including nutrition, exercise, and mental health.
    - Stay informed about the latest research and developments in areas relevant to your health.

  - **Advocate for Preventive Care:**
    - Promote preventive healthcare measures.
    - Schedule regular checkups and screenings to detect and address potential health issues early.

8. Workplace Advocacy:
  - **Assert Your Needs at Work:**
    - Communicate your needs and concerns in the workplace.
    - Advocate for a healthy work-life balance and reasonable workload.

  - **Address Workplace Stress:**
    - If workplace stressors are affecting your well-being, discuss potential solutions with supervisors or HR.

9. Social Support:
  - **Build a Support System:**
    - Be in the company of a network of friends and family who are there to support you.
    - Share your needs and concerns with those who can provide emotional support.

  - **Community Involvement:**

- Engage in community or support groups related to your interests or challenges.
- Connect with others who share similar experiences.

10. Seek Professional Guidance:
  - **Consult Experts:**
  - When facing complex decisions, seek advice from professionals, whether in health, finance, or personal development.

  - **Legal Support:**
  - In certain situations, consider seeking legal advice to protect your rights and well-being.

11. Empower Others:
  - **Promote Advocacy in Others:**
  - Encourage others to advocate for their well-being.
  - Share resources and information that empower individuals to take charge of their health.

12. Regular Reflection and Adjustment:
  - **Assess Your Well-Being:**
  - Regularly assess your well-being and adjust your advocacy strategies as needed.
  - Be open to reevaluating priorities and making changes that support your overall wellness.

Advocating for your well-being is an ongoing process that involves self-awareness, effective communication, and proactive decision-making. By

taking an active role in advocating for your needs,
you contribute to a more fulfilling and balanced life.

EMOTIONAL AND PSYCHOLOGICAL CONSIDERATION

Emotional and psychological considerations are integral aspects of overall well-being, influencing how individuals perceive, understand, and respond to their experiences. Here's a detailed explanation of how emotional and psychological factors impact various facets of life:

1. Emotional Intelligence:

   - **Definition:**
     - Emotional intelligence involves recognizing, understanding, and managing one's own emotions and effectively navigating interpersonal relationships.

   - **Impact on Well-Being:**
     - Individuals with high emotional intelligence tend to experience greater emotional well-being, exhibit resilience in the face of challenges, and establish healthier connections with others.

2. Mental Health Awareness:

   - **Stigma Reduction:**

- Promoting mental health awareness helps reduce the stigma associated with mental health conditions.
    - Open conversations and education contribute to a more supportive environment for those facing mental health challenges.

  - **Access to Resources:**
    - Raising awareness ensures individuals have access to mental health resources and support services.
    - This empowers them to seek help when needed and fosters a culture of understanding.

3. Stress Management:

  - **Impact on Physical Health:**
    - Chronic stress can negatively affect physical health. Emotional and psychological well-being is closely tied to stress management.
    - Adopting effective coping mechanisms, such as mindfulness or relaxation techniques, contributes to overall well-being.

4. Coping Mechanisms:

  - **Healthy Coping Strategies:**
    - Developing healthy coping mechanisms is crucial for emotional resilience.
    - Individuals who employ positive coping strategies, such as seeking social support,

engaging in hobbies, or practicing self-care, are better equipped to manage life's challenges.

5. Trauma-Informed Approaches:

   - **Recognition of Trauma:**
     - A trauma-informed approach acknowledges the impact of past traumas on an individual's emotional and psychological well-being.
     - It focuses on creating environments that prioritize safety, trust, and empowerment.

   - **Supportive Interventions:**
     - Trauma-informed interventions aim to provide support and avoid re-traumatization.
     - Mental health professionals and educators adopting trauma-informed practices create spaces conducive to healing.

6. Relationships and Social Support:

   - **Quality of Relationships:**
     - The quality of interpersonal relationships significantly influences emotional well-being.
     - Nurturing positive connections and seeking social support during times of stress contribute to psychological resilience.

   - **Loneliness and Isolation:**
     - Feelings of loneliness and isolation can have adverse effects on mental health.

- Recognizing the importance of social
connections and addressing feelings of isolation is
vital for emotional well-being.

7. Identity and Self-Perception:

  - **Impact on Self-Esteem:**
    - How individuals perceive themselves and their
sense of identity directly influences their
self-esteem and emotional state.
    - Promoting positive self-perception contributes
to improved psychological well-being.

  - **Cultural Competence:**
    - Recognizing and respecting diverse identities
is crucial for psychological well-being.
    - Culturally competent approaches in therapy,
education, and workplaces enhance understanding
and support.

8. Positive Psychology:

  - **Focus on Strengths:**
    - Positive psychology emphasizes focusing on
individuals' strengths rather than solely addressing
deficits or challenges.
    - Encouraging individuals to leverage their
strengths promotes a more optimistic and resilient
mindset.

9. Cognitive Behavioral Approaches:

- **Cognitive Restructuring:**
    - Cognitive behavioral approaches involve identifying and challenging negative thought patterns.
    - Restructuring cognitive processes contributes to improved emotional regulation and mental well-being.

  - **Behavioral Activation:**
    - Encouraging positive behaviors through behavioral activation is a therapeutic approach to alleviate symptoms of depression and enhance emotional functioning.

10. Seeking Professional Help:

  - **Therapeutic Support:**
    - Seeking professional help when facing emotional or psychological challenges is a proactive step toward well-being.
    - Therapeutic interventions, such as counseling or psychotherapy, provide individuals with tools to navigate their emotions and improve mental health.

11. Self-Reflection and Mindfulness:

  - **Mindfulness Practices:**
    - Incorporating mindfulness practices, such as meditation or deep breathing exercises, supports emotional regulation and stress reduction.
    - Self-reflection enhances self-awareness and facilitates personal growth.

12. Holistic Approach:

   - **Integration of Factors:**
     - A holistic approach to emotional and psychological well-being recognizes the interconnectedness of physical, emotional, and mental health.
     - Addressing these factors collectively contributes to a more comprehensive sense of well-being.

In conclusion, emotional and psychological considerations are fundamental to a person's overall well-being. By fostering emotional intelligence, promoting mental health awareness, and adopting supportive approaches, individuals can cultivate resilience and navigate life's challenges more effectively. Seeking professional help when needed and embracing a holistic perspective contribute to a balanced and thriving emotional and psychological state.

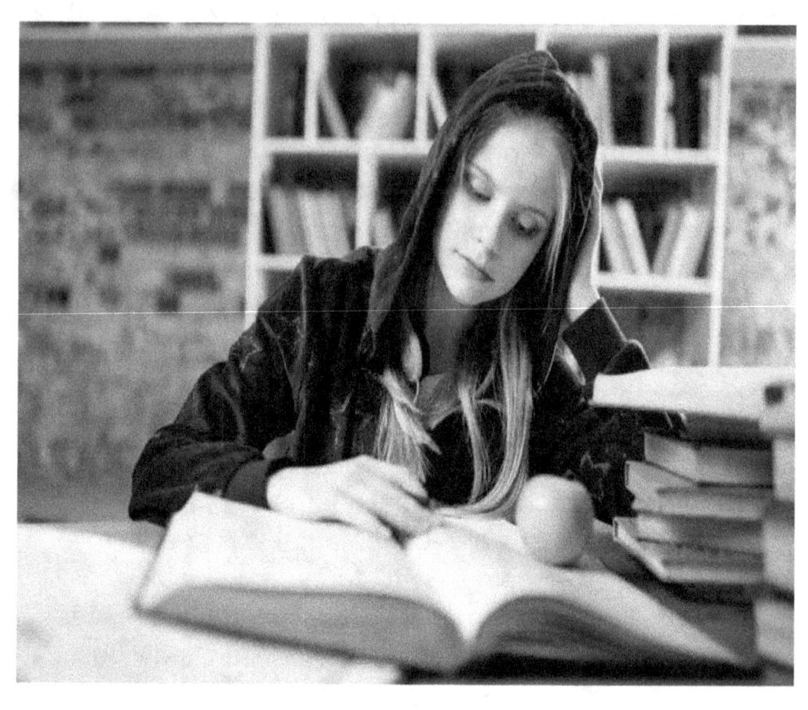

CONCLUSION

In conclusion, taking charge of your fertility is a transformative journey that involves a deep understanding of your body, proactive decision-making, and a commitment to overall reproductive well-being. By delving into the intricacies of your menstrual cycle, embracing fertility awareness methods, and utilizing tools like charting, basal body temperature monitoring, and ovulation prediction kits, you empower yourself with knowledge.

Recognizing the factors that affect fertility, from lifestyle and nutrition to stress management, allows for informed choices that contribute to reproductive health. Addressing common health issues, exploring contraception options, and understanding natural, barrier, and medical methods provide a comprehensive toolkit for navigating fertility choices.

The journey also involves the pursuit of pregnancy, with a focus on timing intercourse for conception, maximizing fertility potential, and troubleshooting challenges that may arise. By actively participating in your reproductive health, you not only enhance your chances of conception but also cultivate a sense of agency and control over this aspect of your life.

In this holistic approach, the recognition of signs of ovulation, understanding the fertile and infertile phases, and addressing irregular cycles become integral components. Seeking professional advice when needed, advocating for your well-being, and acknowledging the emotional and psychological dimensions of fertility contribute to a well-rounded and empowered perspective.

Ultimately, taking charge of your fertility is a dynamic and personalized journey. It involves continuous learning, self-reflection, and adaptation to the evolving needs of your reproductive health. By embracing this proactive approach, individuals not only enhance their chances of achieving their family planning goals but also cultivate a deeper connection with their bodies and a greater sense of control over their reproductive destinies.

TAKING CONTROL OF YOUR FERTILITY JOURNEY

Taking control of your fertility journey is a proactive and empowering endeavor that involves several key steps and considerations. Here's a guide to navigating and taking charge of your fertility journey:

1. Understanding Your Menstrual Cycle:

- Educate yourself about the phases of the menstrual cycle, including menstruation, follicular phase, ovulation, and luteal phase.
- Track your menstrual cycles to identify patterns and estimate the length of your cycle.

2. Basics of Fertility Awareness:
- Familiarize yourself with fertility awareness methods, including tracking menstrual cycles, monitoring basal body temperature (BBT), and observing cervical mucus changes.

3. Charting Your Cycle:
- Use a fertility chart to record important data about your menstrual cycle, including the start and end of menstruation, changes in cervical mucus, and any observed physical symptoms.

4. Recording Basal Body Temperature (BBT):
- Before getting out of bed every morning, measure your BBT. A slight increase in BBT typically indicates ovulation, helping you identify your fertile window.

5. Monitoring Cervical Mucus:
- Observe how your cervical mucus varies over the course of your cycle. Fertile cervical mucus is clear, slippery, and stretchy – a sign that ovulation is approaching.

6. Using Ovulation Prediction Kits (OPKs):

- Consider incorporating OPKs into your routine
to detect the surge in luteinizing hormone (LH) that
precedes ovulation, helping you pinpoint your fertile
days.

7. Interpreting Your Charts:
- Learn how to interpret your fertility charts to
identify patterns, pinpoint ovulation, and understand
the variations in your menstrual cycle.

8. Identifying Fertile and Infertile Phases:
- Utilize the information gathered from charting,
BBT, and other fertility awareness methods to
distinguish between fertile and infertile phases in
your cycle.

9. Recognizing Signs of Ovulation:
- Be attuned to physical signs of ovulation, such
as mild pelvic pain (mittelschmerz), heightened
sense of smell, and changes in cervical position.

10. Factors Affecting Fertility:
- Understand lifestyle factors that can impact
fertility, including diet, exercise, sleep, and
exposure to environmental toxins.

11. Lifestyle and Nutrition:
- Adopt a healthy lifestyle, including a balanced
diet, regular exercise, and sufficient sleep, to
support overall reproductive health.

12. Stress and Impact:

- Manage stress through relaxation techniques,
meditation, or activities that promote emotional
well-being, as chronic stress can affect fertility.

13. Common Health Issues:
   - Address any underlying health issues that may
affect fertility, such as polycystic ovary syndrome
(PCOS), endometriosis, or thyroid disorders.

14. Contraception Options:
   - Explore contraception options and choose a
method that aligns with your family planning goals.
Be aware of the impact of contraceptives on your
fertility when planning for the future.

15. Natural Methods:
   - Consider natural methods of contraception,
such as fertility awareness-based methods, if you
prefer non-hormonal options.

16. Barrier Method:
   - Understand and utilize barrier methods of
contraception, such as condoms, to prevent
pregnancy while maintaining fertility awareness.

17. Medical Options:
   - Explore medical options if needed, such as
hormonal contraceptives or fertility treatments,
under the guidance of healthcare professionals.

18. Achieving Pregnancy:

- When ready to conceive, time intercourse strategically during the fertile window identified through fertility awareness methods.

19. Timing Intercourse for Conception:
   - Maximize your chances of conception by timing intercourse around your ovulation period, increasing the likelihood of sperm meeting the egg.

20. Maximizing Fertility Potential:
   - Continue to prioritize a healthy lifestyle, manage stress, and monitor your fertility signs to maximize your overall fertility potential.

21. Troubleshooting:
   - If facing challenges or concerns, seek professional advice from reproductive health specialists. Consider a thorough evaluation to identify potential issues and explore appropriate interventions.

22. Addressing Irregular Cycles:
   - If experiencing irregular cycles, work with healthcare professionals to identify underlying causes and implement strategies to regulate your menstrual cycle.

Taking control of your fertility journey involves a combination of knowledge, self-awareness, and proactive decision-making. By integrating these steps into your lifestyle and being attuned to your body's signals, you empower yourself to navigate the complexities of fertility with confidence and informed choices. Remember, every fertility journey is unique, and seeking professional guidance can provide personalized insights tailored to your specific needs and goals.

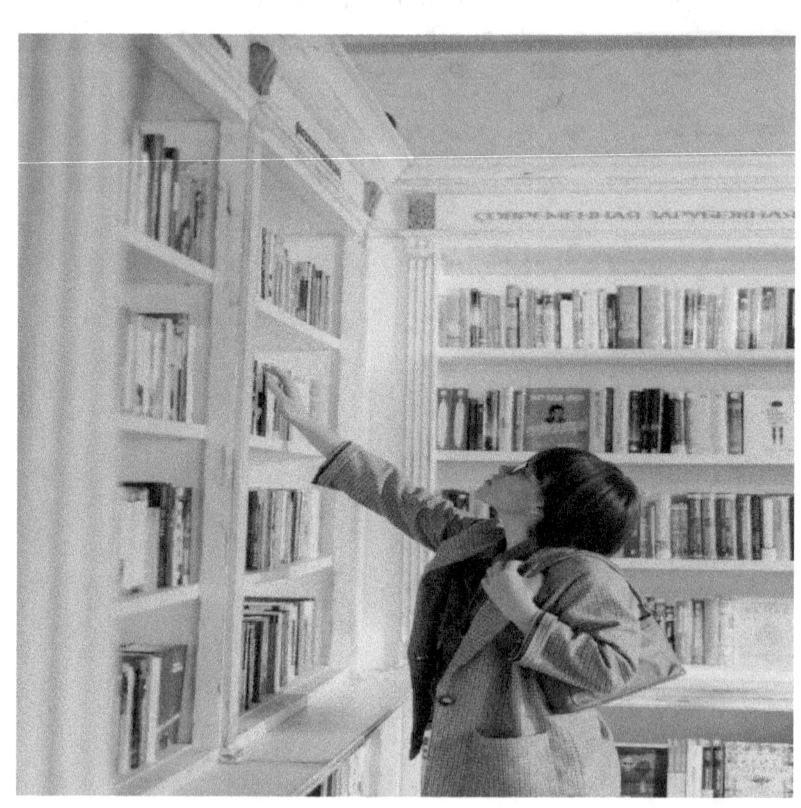

www.ingramcontent.com/pod-product-compliance
Lightning Source LLC
Chambersburg PA
CBHW070811260726
48660CB00005B/1809